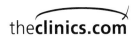
theclinics.com

CLINICS IN PERINATOLOGY

Medical Legal Issues in Perinatal Medicine: Part II

GUEST EDITORS
Isaac Blickstein, MD
Judith L. Chervenak, MD, JD
Frank A. Chervenak, MD

September 2007 • Volume 34 • Number 3

SAUNDERS

An Imprint of Elsevier, Inc.
PHILADELPHIA   LONDON   TORONTO   MONTREAL   SYDNEY   TOKYO

W.B. SAUNDERS COMPANY
A Division of Elsevier Inc.

Elsevier, Inc., 1600 John F. Kennedy Blvd., Suite 1800, Philadelphia, PA 19103-2899

http://www.theclinics.com

CLINICS IN PERINATOLOGY
September 2007
Editor: Carla Holloway

Volume 34, Number 3
ISSN 0095-5108
ISBN-10: 1-4160-5482-0
ISBN-13: 978-1-4160-5482-5

Reprints. For copies of 100 or more of articles in this publication, please contact the commercial Reprints Department, Elsevier Inc., 360 Park Avenue South, New York, New York 10010-1710. Tel: (212) 633-3813 Fax: (212) 462-1935, e-mail: reprints@elsevier.com.

The ideas and opinions expressed in *Clinics in Perinatology* do not necessarily reflect those of the Publisher. The Publisher does not assume any responsibility for any injury and/or damage to persons or property arising out of or related to any use of the material contained in this periodical. The reader is advised to check the appropriate medical literature and the product information currently provided by the manufacturer of each drug to be administered, to verify the dosage, the method and duration of administration or contraindications. It is the responsibility of the treating physician or other health care professional, relying on independent experience and knowledge of the patient, to determine drug dosages and the best treatment for the patient. Mention of any product in this issue should not be construed as endorsement by the contributors, editors, or the Publisher of the product or manufacturers' claims.

Clinics in Perinatology (ISSN 0095-5108) is published in quarterly by Elsevier Inc., 360 Park Avenue South, New York, NY 10010-1710. Months of issue are March, June, September, and December. Business and Editorial offices: 1600 John F. Kennedy Blvd., Suite 1800, Philadelphia, PA 19103-2899. Customer Service Office: 6277 Sea Harbor Drive, Orlando, FL 32887-4800. Periodicals postage paid at New York, NY and additional mailing offices. Subscription prices are $182.00 per year for (US individuals), $270.00 per year for (US institutions), $215.00 per year (Canadian individuals), $335.00 per year (Canadian institutions), $248.00 per year (foreign individuals), $335.00 per year (foreign institutions) $88.00 per year (US students), and $121.00 per year (foreign students). Foreign air speed delivery is included in all Clinics subscription prices. All prices are subject to change without notice. **POSTMASTER:** Send address changes to *Clinics in Perinatology;* Elsevier Periodicals Customer Service, 6277 Sea Harbor Drive, Orlando, FL 32887-4800. **Customer Service: 1-800-654-2452 (US). From outside of the US, call 1-407-345-1000.** E-mail: elspcs@elsevier.com

Clinics in Perinatology is also pubilshed in Spanish by McGraw-Hill Interamericana Editores S.A., P.O. Box 5-237, 06500 Mexico D.F., Mexico.

Clinics in Perinatology is covered in *Index Medicus, Current Contents, Excepta Medica, BIOSIS* and *ISI/BIOMED.*

Printed in the United States of America.

GUEST EDITORS

ISAAC BLICKSTEIN, MD, Department of Obstetrics and Gynecology, Kaplan Medical Center, Rehovot; Hadassah-Hebrew University School of Medicine, Jerusalem, Israel

JUDITH L. CHERVENAK, MD, JD, Clinical Assistant Professor of Obstetrics and Gynecology, New York University School of Medicine; of Counsel, Heidell, Pittoni, Murphy & Bach, LLP, New York, New York

FRANK A. CHERVENAK, MD, Given Foundation Professor and Chairman; Obstetrician; Gynecologist-in-Chief, Department of Obstetrics and Gynecology, Joan and Sanford I. Weill Medical College of Cornell University, The New York Presbyterian Hospital, New York, New York

CONTRIBUTORS

ROBERT H. ALLEN, PhD, Associate Research Professor, Department of Biomedical Engineering, The Johns Hopkins University, Baltimore, Maryland

EROL AMON, MD, JD, Professor and Director of Maternal-Fetal Medicine, Department of Obstetrics, Gynecology, and Women's Health, Saint Louis University, St. Louis, Missouri

REBECCA N. BAERGEN, MD, Professor of Clinical Pathology and Laboratory Medicine; Chief of Perinatal and Pediatric Pathology, New York Presbyterian Hospital, Weill-Cornell Medical Center, Department of Pathology, New York, New York

ISAAC BLICKSTEIN, MD, Department of Obstetrics and Gynecology, Kaplan Medical Center, Rehovot; Hadassah-Hebrew University School of Medicine, Jerusalem, Israel

FRANK A. CHERVENAK, MD, Given Foundation Professor and Chairman; Obstetrician; Gynecologist-in-Chief, Department of Obstetrics and Gynecology, Joan and Sanford I. Weill Medical College of Cornell University, The New York Presbyterian Hospital, New York, New York

ORNA FLIDEL-RIMON, MD, Department of Neonatology, Kaplan Medical Center, Rehovot; Hebrew University, Jerusalem, Israel

TAMAR GREEN, MD, Department of Obstetrics and Gynecology, Kaplan Medical Center, Rehovot, Israel

AMOS GRUNEBAUM, MD, Director of Obstetrics; Chief of Labor and Delivery; Assistant Professor of Obstetrics and Gynecology, New York Weill Cornell Medical College, New York, New York

EDITH D. GUREWITSCH, MD, Assistant Professor, Department of Gynecology/Obstetrics, Division of Maternal Fetal Medicine, The Johns Hopkins University School of Medicine, The Johns Hopkins Hospital; Department of Biomedical Engineering, The Johns Hopkins University, Baltimore, Maryland

LISA M. KORST, MD, PhD, Associate Professor, Department of Obstetrics and Gynecology, USC Keck School of Medicine, North Hollywood, California

GILBERT I. MARTIN, MD, Clinical Professor; Director of Neonatal Services, Citrus Valley Medical Center, University of California Irvine, West Covina, California

LAURENCE B. MCCULLOUGH, PhD, Center for Medical Ethics and Health Policy, Baylor College of Medicine, Houston, Texas

JEFFREY P. PHELAN, MD, JD, Vice Chairman and Director of Quality Assurance, Department of Obstetrics and Gynecology, Citrus Valley Medical Center, West Covina, California

STEVEN F. SEIDMAN, MD, JD, Of Counsel, Heidell, Pittoni, Murphy & Bach, LLP, New York, New York

ERIC STUART SHINWELL, MD, Department of Neonatology, Kaplan Medical Center, Rehovot; Hebrew University, Jerusalem, Israel

HUNG N. WINN, MD, JD, MBA, David G. Hall Professor of Obstetrics and Gynecology; Chairman, Department of Obstetrics, Gynecology and Women's Health, University of Missouri-Columbia School of Medicine, Columbia, Missouri

CONTENTS

Using an evidence-based, medical approach, the strengths and
pitfalls of the causation- and standard-of-care–based arguments
proffered by plaintiff and defense counsel in shoulder dystocia–
associated birth injury litigation are reviewed based on medical
plausibility. The role of the expert witness as arbiter of the relationship between medical care rendered and the untoward outcome
of such care is distinguished from that of other court members.
Proposed solutions to the medical malpractice litigation crisis are
also examined in light of relevant differences in the pathogenetic
bases for birth injuries of various types.

Group B streptococcus (*streptococcus agalactiae*), a gram-positive
coccus, is one of the major causes of maternal or neonatal severe
infection and sepsis. Maternal infection associated with GBS
includes acute chorioamnionitis, endometritis, and urinary tract
infection.

The placenta not only "records" and reflects the intrauterine environment, it also provides valuable information on the cause and
timing of many adverse events and conditions. The placenta may
be useful in several ways. It may be the cause of injury due to an
inherent abnormality, it may "malfunction" because of disease

processes that are not primarily placental in origin, or it may merely reflect an abnormal intrauterine environment. Not only may the etiology of the injury be ascertained from placental examination, but also a time frame during which the abnormal condition has been operating. Acute lesions may be associated with sudden catastrophic events, whereas other, more chronic lesions lead to decreased placental reserves. Markedly depleted reserves will render the infant susceptible to other, sometimes more acute, events and thus are also associated with significant injury or even death.

The purpose of this article is to familiarize the reader with the concept of causation and the role of the concept of foreseeability of harm in obstetric malpractice lawsuits. These concepts are incorporated into several hypothetical fetal brain injury and uterine rupture cases. The discussion involves an overview of available scientific evidence used to substantiate or refute whether a child's brain damage or a maternal uterine rupture was in fact related to the obstetric care in question. In the event of the delivery of a depressed newborn, a checklist of scientific evidence to be gathered at the time of delivery is also provided.

Recent years have witnessed an international, multisource effort to define and progressively improve evidence-based criteria for defining the relationship between perinatal events and the subsequent development of cerebral palsy. The neonatal components of these criteria include neonatal encephalopathy, Apgar score, multisystem organ dysfunction, and currently available neuroimaging methods. This review focuses on current knowledge and unresolved issues regarding these criteria.

The intrapartum acid-base status of the fetus is an important component in establishing the link between intrapartum events and neonatal condition. The analysis of cord blood gases from the umbilical artery is believed to be the best representation of the fetal acid-base status immediately before birth. Blood gas analysis is able to objectively confirm or exclude the presence of damaging acidemia. Although measurements may be affected by several factors related to the method of sampling, storage, and assessment, a wide margin of accuracy exists when prompt assessment is unavailable. Because a substantial deviation from the standard procedure is required before a sample is alleged to be imprecise, it is unlikely that standard sampling methods would be ineligible in litigation.

Quality medical care focuses on achieving the greatest benefit while minimizing the risk of patient harm. This standard can become clouded in the case of a parturient and her fetus. The maternal–fetal relationship is unlike any other faced by physicians due to the fetus' complete physiologic dependence on the mother and because both the fetus and mother are considered patients of the obstetrician. This article reviews the ethical principles in obstetrics and gynecology and the laws and regulations that define professional misconduct. Although professional misconduct and ethics are separate entities, there are times when a physician's conduct must be examined from the standpoint of statutory misconduct and ethical uncertainties.

One of the most important interfaces between medicine and law occurs in the courtroom. When medical issues are litigated, physicians have potential to make excellent witnesses. This article reviews the proper role, qualifications, and ethical requirements of expert witnesses, the law of professional negligence, and the regulation of unprofessional testimony. Expert witness reform is also briefly discussed.

This article outlines an approach to improve patient safety in obstetrics and gynecology, with the goal to reduce errors in labor and delivery. Every institution should create guidelines and provide education and training to address potential safety issues such as fetal heart rate pattern interpretation, induction and stimulation of labor, vaginal birth after cesarean, magnesium sulfate, shoulder dystocia, hemorrhage, forceps/vacuum, and thromboembolic disease. This article discusses the patient safety objectives published by the American College of Obstetricians and Gynecologists

Committee on Quality Improvement and Patient Safety; the National Patient Safety Goals, which are regularly established by the Joint Committee on Accreditation of Healthcare Organizations; and patient safety indicators developed by the Agency for Healthcare Research and Quality

The obstetrics–gynecology profession is in the midst of a professional liability crisis. Solutions must come from both individual practitioners and managers/policymakers. The purpose of this article is to provide readers with preventive ethics tools to respond professionally in their own practices to neglected ethical dimensions of the professional liability crisis. The authors' analysis and proposals are based on previous work.

GOAL STATEMENT
The goal of *Clinics in Perinatology* is to keep practicing neonatologists and maternal-fetal medicine specialists up to date with current clinical practice in perinatology by providing timely articles reviewing the state of the art in patient care.

ACCREDITATION
The *Clinics in Perinatology* is planned and implemented in accordance with the Essential Areas and Policies of the Accreditation Council for Continuing Medical Education (ACCME) through the joint sponsorship of the University of Virginia School of Medicine and Elsevier. The University of Virginia School of Medicine is accredited by the ACCME to provide continuing medical education for physicians.

The University of Virginia School of Medicine designates this educational activity for a maximum of 60 *AMA PRA Category 1 Credits*™. Physicians should only claim credit commensurate with the extent of their participation in the activity.

The American Medical Association has determined that physicians not licensed in the US who participate in this CME activity are eligible for *AMA PRA Category 1 Credits*™.

Credit can be earned by reading the text material, taking the CME examination online at http://www.theclinics.com/home/cme, and completing the evaluation. After taking the test, you will be required to review any and all incorrect answers. Following completion of the test and evaluation, your credit will be awarded and you may print your certificate.

FACULTY DISCLOSURE/CONFLICT OF INTEREST
The University of Virginia School of Medicine, as an ACCME accredited provider, endorses and strives to comply with the Accreditation Council for Continuing Medical Education (ACCME) Standards of Commercial Support, Commonwealth of Virginia statutes, University of Virginia policies and procedures, and associated federal and private regulations and guidelines on the need for disclosure and monitoring of proprietary and financial interests that may affect the scientific integrity and balance of content delivered in continuing medical education activities under our auspices.

The University of Virginia School of Medicine requires that all CME activities accredited through this institution be developed independently and be scientifically rigorous, balanced and objective in the presentation/discussion of its content, theories and practices.

All authors/editors participating in an accredited CME activity are expected to disclose to the readers relevant financial relationships with commercial entities occurring within the past 12 months (such as grants or research support, employee, consultant, stock holder, member of speakers bureau, etc.). The University of Virginia School of Medicine will employ appropriate mechanisms to resolve potential conflicts of interest to maintain the standards of fair and balanced education to the reader. Questions about specific strategies can be directed to the Office of Continuing Medical Education, University of Virginia School of Medicine, Charlottesville, Virginia.

The authors/editors listed below have identified no professional or financial affiliations for themselves or their spouse/partner:
Robert H. Allen, PhD; Rebecca N. Baergen, MD; Isaac Blickstein, MD (Guest Editor); Frank A. Chervenak, MD (Guest Editor); Judith L. Chervenak, MD, JD (Guest Editor); Orna Flidel-Rimon, MD; Tamar Green, MD; Amos Grunebaum, MD; Carla Holloway (Acquisitions Editor); Lisa M. Korst, MD, PhD; Gilbert I. Martin, MD; Laurence B. McCullough, PhD; Jeffrey P. Phelan, MD, JD; Eric Stuart Shinwell, MD; and Hung N. Winn, MD, JD, MBA.

The authors/editors listed below identified the following professional or financial affiliations for themselves or their spouse/partner:
Erol Amon, MD, JD owns stock in Johnson & Johnson and Sonosite, and is an independent contractor for Protherics.
Edith D. Gurewitsch, MD has received grants for Biomechanics Traumatic Injuries Research from CDC/NCIPC, and is on the advisory committee/board of CDC/NCIPC.
Steven F. Seidman, MD, JD owns stock in Amgen, Glaxo-Smith Kline, and Boston Life Science.

Disclosure of Discussion of non-FDA approved uses for pharmaceutical products and/or medical devices:
The University of Virginia School of Medicine, as an ACCME provider, requires that all faculty presenters identify and disclose any "off label" uses for pharmaceutical and medical device products. The University of Virginia School of Medicine recommends that each physician fully review all the available data on new products or procedures prior to instituting them with patients.

TO ENROLL
To enroll in the Clinics in Perinatology Continuing Medical Education program, call customer service at 1-800-654-2452 or visit us online at www.theclinics.com/home/cme. The CME program is available to subscribers for an additional fee of $195.00.

FORTHCOMING ISSUES

Iatrogenic Disease
Marcus Hermansen, MD, *Guest Editor*

Cesarean Section
Lucky Jain, MD
Ronald Wapner, MD, *Guest Editors*

Neuroprotection in the High-Risk Newborn
Alan R. Spitzer, MD
Robert D. White, *Guest Editors*

RECENT ISSUES

June 2007
Medical Legal Issues in Perinatal Medicine: Part I
Isaac Blickstein, MD
Judith Chervenak, MD, JD
Frank Chervenak, MD, *Guest Editors*

March 2007
Surfactant and Mechanical Ventilation
Steven M. Donn, MD
Thomas E. Wiswell, MD, *Guest Editors*

December 2006
Late Preterm Pregnancy and the Newborn
Lucky Jain, MD, MBA
Tonse N.K. Raju, MD, DCH, *Guest Editors*

Preface

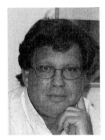

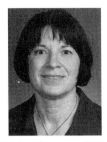

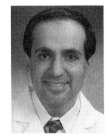

Isaac Blickstein, MD   Judith L. Chervenak, MD, JD   Frank A. Chervenak, MD

Guest Editors

The definition of medical malpractice is an act or omission by a health care provider that deviates from accepted standards of practice in the medical community and that causes injury to the patient. The specialty of perinatal medicine is among the top-ranking disciplines associated with malpractice claims in most developed countries. Perhaps the primary reason is that, by default, any pregnant woman expects to have a perfect child and to step out of the delivery room as healthy as she was before pregnancy. However, pregnancy and childbirth are essentially risky. When the maternal expectation does not concur with professional reality, dispute may arise. In addition, the overabundance of technology associated with prenatal diagnosis and the amount of sophistication available in perinatal medicine have led to the wrong popular perception of omnipotence. Often, a deviation from the expected perfect outcome is assumed to be a consequence of negligence.

As a result, the 2003 Annual Report from the National Practitioner Data Bank indicates that 16,764 medical malpractice payments were made due to obstetrics-related malpractice by physicians in the United States 1990 to 2003, with a mean and median medical malpractice payment due to obstetrics-related malpractice of $377,305 and $200,000, respectively. According to the same source, payments increased over the years, and among the 1255 medical malpractice payments made due to obstetrics-related malpractice in the United States 2003, the mean and median medical malpractice

doi:10.1016/j.clp.2007.07.001   *perinatology.theclinics.com*

payment due to obstetrics-related malpractice were \$475,880 and \$290,000, respectively. In total, \$2,824,280,036 in payments was made for obstetrics-related primary malpractice acts or omissions in the United States 1990 to 1996.

These facts translate to increased malpractice insurance premiums, which in turn, have the potential to decrease future availability of specialist services. Despite these downsides, tort claims have a definite educational role by identifying weak points that need improvement and teaching the medical community about how to avoid negligence. On top of everything are lawyers who seek to provide compensation for damages occurring during the perinatal period because of alleged malpractice and negligence or to defend clinicians against such allegations. Collectively, the current medicolegal environment presents significant challenges to clinicians and lawyers.

In most lawsuits, cases with or without clear-cut malpractice are easily recognized. The problem is the "gray zone," which is unfortunately common in perinatal medicine. With these points in mind, our intention was neither to rewrite textbooks in perinatal medicine nor to provide guidelines for clinical practice. Instead, we wanted to identify and discuss the most common clinical situations that lead to legal disputes related to perinatal medicine to delineate the "gray zone," to focus on controversies, and to provide the contrasting perspective related to how a clinical situation is perceived by the practitioner and by the lawyer.

This issue is the second part of *Clinics in Perinatology* devoted to an interdisciplinary discussion on medicolegal issues in perinatal medicine. In this part, readers may find in-depth considerations of causation, as well as extended commentaries related to the alleged association between an intrapartum event and development of cerebral palsy. Relevant ethical issues are also discussed.

The editors wish to thank all authors for the scholarly contributions and to Mrs. Carla Holloway—the production manager of this issue—for her continuous help and support.

Isaac Blickstein, MD
Department of Obstetrics and Gynecology
Kaplan Medical Center
76100 Rehovot, Israel

Hadassah-Hebrew University School of Medicine
Jerusalem, Israel

E-mail address: blick@netvision.net.il

Judith L. Chervenak, MD, JD
Heidell, Pittoni, Murphy & Bach, LLP
99 Park Avenue
New York, NY 10016, USA

New York University School of Medicine
550 First Avenue
New York, NY 10016, USA

E-mail address: jchervenak@hpmb.com

Frank A. Chervenak, MD
Department of Obstetrics and Gynecology
Joan and Sanford I. Weill Medical College of Cornell University
The New York Presbyterian Hospital
525 East 68th Street, Box 122
New York, NY 10021, USA

E-mail address: fac2001@med.cornell.edu

ELSEVIER
SAUNDERS

CLINICS IN
PERINATOLOGY

Clin Perinatol 34 (2007) 365–385

Shoulder Dystocia

Edith D. Gurewitsch, MD[a,b,*], Robert H. Allen, PhD[b]

[a]Department of Gynecology/Obstetrics, Division of Maternal Fetal Medicine,
The Johns Hopkins University School of Medicine, The Johns Hopkins Hospital,
600 North Wolfe Street – Phipps 217, Baltimore, MD 21287, USA
[b]Department of Biomedical Engineering, The Johns Hopkins University,
3400 North Charles Street, Clark Hall 118-C, Baltimore, MD 21218, USA

Brachial plexus injury following shoulder dystocia is the third most common cause for litigation within obstetrics [1], accounting for nearly 11% of lawsuits filed in that discipline [2,3]. Among malpractice cases involving birth injury, brachial plexus palsy (which can also occur in non-cephalic, non–shoulder dystocia deliveries [4]) ranks second only to peripartum hypoxic ischemic encephalopathy [5], which itself is another potential untoward outcome of shoulder dystocia (although far less common) that may also prompt legal action by parents on behalf of their minor child. Rarely, allegations of malpractice leading to permanent sequelae from maternal injuries incurred during shoulder dystocia can also find their way into a courtroom [6].

A harrowing experience for clinician and patient alike, shoulder dystocia deliveries that are complicated by injury are fraught with myriad emotional responses on both sides, including bewilderment, denial, anger, and guilt. Each party can emerge from the event with more questions than answers, leading to dissatisfying clinician–patient encounters. The patient's growing suspicion of clinician neglect or misconduct is met with the clinician's defensiveness and counteraccusations of patient noncompliance. Fueling this conflagration are the difficulties in prognosticating about expected recovery in the immediate aftermath of the delivery and that clinical follow-up most often will not be occurring with the original health care team, especially not with the obstetric provider.

Much has been written about the need for honest, cautious, sympathetic, consistent, and ongoing communication between clinician and patient

* Corresponding author. Department of Gynecology/Obstetrics, Division of Maternal Fetal Medicine, The Johns Hopkins Hospital, 600 North Wolfe Street – Phipps 217, Baltimore, Maryland 21287.
E-mail address: egurewi@jhmi.edu (E.D. Gurewitsch).

perinatology.theclinics.com

following a shoulder dystocia delivery that was complicated by injury and other adverse events [7–13]. Communication of all types (eg, clinician-to-patient, clinician-to-clinician, and clinician-to-hospital administration) is the best method by which to gain a better understanding of therapeutic goals and expectations, improve crisis resource management, and avert litigation. Certainly, reducing the incidence of the untoward outcomes themselves also reduces the incidence of shoulder dystocia–related malpractice claims [14]. This latter strategy is best accomplished by way of continued practice-based medical education, quality improvement reviews, competency assessment, and rehearsal drills. Ongoing research into mechanisms of injury and optimal management of shoulder dystocia to mitigate permanence and severity of injury is of paramount importance [15,16]. All these topics are beyond the scope of this article, however. The premise of this article is that a shoulder dystocia–associated permanent birth injury has occurred and legal action already has been initiated against the obstetric provider.

The authors of this paper are academicians, not attorneys. Through our professional collaboration, we have between us decades of clinical and research expertise in the area of shoulder dystocia and its related injuries. Independently, we each have been invited by both plaintiff and defense to review many cases of shoulder dystocia–associated birth injury that are in a various stages of litigation, from initial risk-management review or determination of merit before suit is filed to rebuttal of expert opinions already rendered during testimony given in ongoing cases. With review of each such case, we continue to learn from clinical examples of shoulder dystocia–associated birth injury that would not otherwise be accessible to us or be amassed in a database collection that could be explored.[1] From this effort, we are able to develop and test hypotheses that can be studied experimentally and our results can then be disseminated to the medical community [17–21]. We are committed first and foremost to objectivity. This objectivity is imperative not only to the integrity of our research but also to the charge we are given for our expert reviews: to judge impartially the relationship between medical care that was rendered and the outcome derived. Impartiality is precisely the stance we adopt in the following review of the medicolegal issues that arise in shoulder dystocia–associated birth injury cases. It is the aim of this paper to evaluate objectively the strength of existing evidentiary support for plaintiff allegations and defense arguments based on available research and practice guidelines.

---

[1] Our research activity derived from review of litigated cases has approval from the Institutional Review Board of the Johns Hopkins Medical Institutions. To avoid conflict of interest and to protect the privacy and interests of all parties to ongoing litigation, the anonymous data we amass, review, and collectively analyze from legal cases are entered into our research database only after each litigated case has been formally closed (ie, dismissed, settled or verdict has been rendered).

Standard of care and causation

The perspective of the expert witness

In malpractice litigation there are two issues that must be decided by the judge and jury: First, was the standard of care breached? And second, did a breach of the standard of care, if it occurred, contribute to or cause the injury? Unless both questions are answered in the affirmative, based on a preponderance of the evidence, there cannot be a finding of liability. For the expert witness, however, these issues are not necessarily (indeed, often they are not) mutually determinative. As "persons in possession of greater knowledge than the general population about a particular subject or discipline," expert witnesses have a professional duty to relate the facts of a case to those aspects of standard of care and causation that can be known or would be most plausible within the context of their discipline. To do so, expert witnesses draw on their education, training, experience, and familiarity with the relevant scientific bases for theories put forth by either side. It should be neither the aim nor the responsibility of the expert witness to frame the legal strategy for the counselors in the case. Realistically, experts often have to make concessions to the opposing side, because it is rare that all aspects of care were substandard or that each substandard practice they identify is relevant as a proximate cause of the injury in the case. Likewise, even if a clinician's actions were most likely to have been the direct cause of an injury, not all such actions would necessarily fall below the standard of care. It is the function of the expert witness to educate the court members about such distinctions.

Not infrequently, counsel for either side attempts to reduce the arguments in a case to absolutes, leaving the jury to contend with deciding between equally unlikely claims: either the injury was entirely avoidable had the correct management been used or the injury bears no relationship to anything the obstetric provider did or did not do. Often the available evidence in the literature is contorted to fit such arguments, leading to persistent misinterpretations of incidences of particular types of injuries and blurred distinctions between clinically relevant and irrelevant injuries and their respective pathogeneses. Limitations of study design and data analysis are frequently overlooked. Furthermore, attorneys may rely on recently reported scientific results that are based on small samples or even the existence of rare case reports as being conclusive support for their position when these results have yet to be repeated, validated, or proven to have withstood the test of time.

We next take up each of these absolute arguments and consider their fallacies based on available evidence. Thereafter, we proffer our systematic, objective approach to the evaluation of standard of care and causation, recognizing that, in the final analysis, every case must be individualized.

Allegations by plaintiff

Allowing vaginal delivery was negligent: the failure to predict or prevent shoulder dystocia

A compelling argument to jurors is the notion that all delivery complications should be foreseeable and that the vast armamentarium of modern medicine is sufficient to prevent their occurrence altogether. In the case of shoulder dystocia–associated birth injury, the argument usually takes the form of a claim that the shoulder dystocia was destined to happen, that this "fact" was not only knowable but obvious before delivery, and that rightfully it should have been avoided by cesarean delivery, either a priori before labor began or at some point during labor when the inevitability of shoulder dystocia should have become apparent to any reasonable practitioner. The corollary to this argument often surrounds the issue of informed consent: had the woman only been alerted to the possibility of complications with vaginal delivery, such as shoulder dystocia and its associated morbidities, and offered the option of cesarean delivery as an alternative, she naturally would have elected this option. Retrospective studies that identify specific risk factors for shoulder dystocia, such as fetal macrosomia, maternal obesity or diabetes, postdatism, second-stage length abnormalities, and instrumented delivery [22–28], are heavily relied on to buttress the argument that shoulder dystocia can be anticipated. An increase in patient consumerism within medicine and popular abhorrence of paternalistic practice styles that subvert patient autonomy renders the simple suggestion of misconduct on the part of the clinician in failing to invite the patient's full and autonomous participation in her own care usually sufficient to persuade a jury.

From the expert's perspective, the above arguments are hardly as clearcut as plaintiff's counsel would have the court members believe. First, more studies demonstrating a lack of reliability of risk factors as positive predictors of shoulder dystocia occurrence can be proffered as counterargument to the contention that shoulder dystocia was recognizably inevitable [29–36]. What the layperson interpreting the available literature on the subject of risk factors for shoulder dystocia usually fails to realize is the distinction between case-control and cohort study designs. In the former, cases with and without shoulder dystocia are examined retrospectively for differences in the prevalence of certain risk factors between groups; in the latter type of study design, cohorts of women with and without risk factors are prospectively examined to determine differences in the incidence of shoulder dystocia between groups. Although it is fairly common that a given case of shoulder dystocia will, retrospectively, prove to have been associated with several commonly recognized risk factors, it is more likely that any given woman who has certain risk factors will not experience a shoulder dystocia at delivery than that she would.

Second, and more importantly, some of the same risk factors for shoulder dystocia, especially obesity and diabetes, also predispose to significant complications from surgery, such as pulmonary embolism, wound dehiscence, and anesthetic complications. Although intuitive, it is not actually true that simply bypassing vaginal delivery by performing cesarean section averts all possible untoward outcomes associated with birth. Often there is a trade-off between potential maternal morbidity and potential fetal morbidity. Neither is it so that all women necessarily prioritize fetal outcome over maternal outcome if they are in an unenviable position of having to choose between the two. Herein lays the clinical dilemma facing the practitioner planning and managing the labor and delivery of a woman who has significant risk factors for adverse outcome from both shoulder dystocia and cesarean delivery. Far more often, cesarean delivery is performed for fetal indications (ie, specifically to optimize fetal outcome) and not for maternal indications. Under usual circumstances, cesarean section should be performed when the benefit to the fetus of not being born vaginally (eg, when there is fetal distress in labor or malpresentation) far outweighs the risk to the mother of undergoing major abdominal surgery. Because it is the adverse outcome of shoulder dystocia, and not shoulder dystocia itself, that we seek to prevent, and because most shoulder dystocia deliveries do not result in any harm and far fewer actually result in permanent injury, the justification for placing the mother at surgical risk, even when that risk is small, is lacking. When maternal risk is more substantial, as it would be for the very types of women who are also at increased risk for shoulder dystocia, a significant and measurable improvement in fetal outcome over the alternative of a trial of labor becomes primary and imperative before risking maternal morbidity (and even mortality) can be tolerated. The indiscriminate, empiric use of cesarean section in a large population of at-risk mother–infant pairs to avoid the rare permanent brachial plexus injury from shoulder dystocia is especially rash and potentially irresponsible medically and fiscally [34].

It is precisely this conundrum about optimal clinical management of shoulder dystocia risk that led the American College of Obstetrics and Gynecology to revise the estimated fetal weight cut-offs for diabetic and non-diabetic women above which elective primary cesarean section should be raised as a possibility with the at-risk patient to 4500 g and 5000 g, respectively [37]. The standard of care, as articulated in the 2002 Practice Bulletin entitled *Shoulder Dystocia* and remaining in effect today, does not even require consideration of cesarean section below this cut-off. Even above this cut-off, cesarean section is not mandated. Rather, it is first at this point that the standard of care includes bringing the woman's preferences to bear on planning the mode of delivery. Given that the frequency of estimated fetal weights or of actual birth weights that exceed these cut-offs in the general population is <1%, and are still uncommon even among shoulder dystocia births, it is the rare case of shoulder dystocia–associated birth injury in which either the estimated fetal weight or the actual birth weight was such that a failure to offer a cesarean section in the face of recognizable risk factors for shoulder dystocia could even be considered a breach of the standard of care.

Recognizing that most shoulder dystocia–associated brachial plexus injury cases rarely have, even in retrospect, met the indications for prelabor cesarean section, what then can be said about other aspects of the intrapartum management that preceded the shoulder dystocia event, such as the decision to induce labor for fetal macrosomia, to augment labor in the face of a protracted active phase of the first stage, or to shorten the second stage by use of forceps or vacuum? Unfortunately, an examination of the literature on these and other issues yields the same paradox between retrospective case-control and prospective-cohort or even randomized-controlled trials of such management approaches. For example, high birth weight is most decidedly a risk factor for shoulder dystocia, and the extremely high birth weight is among the most consistent (although by no means exclusive) variables that correlate with shoulder dystocia severity and with injury [38,39]. It would therefore makes sense to attempt to ensure lower birth weight through earlier delivery than would otherwise occur if labor were allowed to ensue naturally. The practice of inducing labor for fetal macrosomia has proven ineffective in avoiding or even decreasing the incidence of shoulder dystocia in at-risk maternal–infant dyads and (somewhat counterintuitively) is actually associated with a higher cesarean section rate compared with those expectantly managed [40–42]. Similarly, although instrumented deliveries are, when retrospectively assessed, commonly associated with shoulder dystocia [28,43], and instrumented deliveries in general are more likely to result in fetal or maternal injury compared with spontaneous vaginal deliveries [18,44–46], when prospectively considered most instrumented deliveries are safe and uneventful [47]. Even when intuitive or emotionally compelling, axiomatic approaches to shoulder dystocia prevention (eg, prophylactic McRoberts' maneuver) or management (eg, episiotomy) may prove untenable once subjected to clinical study [20,48].

Critical analysis of the methods and results of the aforementioned studies and of the highly circumscribed or nonspecific policies they necessarily engender yields many opinions about their generalizability and applicability to an individual instance of a shoulder dystocia–associated permanent injury. Questions also can be raised about the advisability of compounding risk factors for shoulder dystocia, such as choosing to perform an operative delivery in an obese woman who has diabetes and is undergoing induction of labor for evidence of accelerated fetal growth. Nevertheless, it is decidedly premature, undoubtedly costly, and potentially dangerous to have the standard of care be determined in the courtroom rather than by rigorous scientific inquiry. The practice of "defensive medicine" to reduce vulnerability to future litigation, although understandable in light of the malpractice litigation crisis in obstetrics that has emerged in recent years, is expensive and not without its own risks of incurring unnecessary testing and interventions that themselves increase the likelihood of complications. In nearly all circumstances in which defensive medicine could be used, there is a balance to be struck between competing clinical issues. Despite the preferences and strategic approaches that a given medical expert, as a representative "reasonably prudent practitioner," would have used in managing an individual at-risk parturient, the same expert must concede that other reasonably prudent practitioners would choose different approaches. Until the superiority and acceptability of one approach over another can be established by a preponderance of scientific evidence, it is unjustified for an expert to levy criticism against an individual practitioner couched in terms of having breached the standard of care for actions (or inactions) that amount to a judgment call.

Res ipsa loquitur: "The injury speaks for itself"

Just as it is compelling to believe that every misadventure in the process of labor and delivery could have been foreseen and forestalled, so too is the notion that if handled properly conditions that may predispose to injury should never actually result in injury. Such is the standard allegation by plaintiffs' attorneys (and many of their experts): The mere existence of a permanent brachial plexus palsy that was present from birth—no matter its extent or classification—necessarily bespeaks negligence or misconduct on the part of the delivering clinician. Whether it was failure to diagnose shoulder dystocia [29] or use of excessive traction during its management [49–51], the critical—indeed the only—determinant of permanent injury, according to the proponents of this argument, had to have been the clinician. Setting aside the facts that there are other non–birth process–related causes of congenital brachial plexus palsy [52] and that temporary brachial plexus injuries occur in the absence of recorded shoulder dystocia [21,24,53] or even traction to the fetal head [54], it is far more common that permanent brachial plexus injuries are the domain of shoulder dystocia–complicated births [21,38,55–59] and it is well established that obstetric brachial plexus injuries are stretch-induced injuries [60–62] readily, although not necessarily exclusively [63], produced by clinician-applied traction [50,51,64–66]. Although this traction was excessive for the injured brachial plexus nerves, it may not have been excessive for delivery. This issue—the conflation of causation with the standard of care—as the allegation of res ipsa loquitur does not have evidentiary support in the available medical literature.

Even when a clinician's actions are likely to be found, by a preponderance of evidence, to have been proximately causative in a shoulder dystocia–associated permanent brachial plexus injury, it does not follow either universally or necessarily that those actions fell beneath the standard of care. A range of traction forces that clinicians apply in various types of deliveries have been measured clinically and experimentally, and demonstrate an expected and necessary increase in the mean of those forces as delivery difficulty increases, especially in shoulder dystocia [51,67–70]. Furthermore, traction of the same magnitude might produce injury in one shoulder dystocia delivery and not in another [51], and biologic variations in brachial plexus anatomy [71] may predispose some infants to injury compared with others. Finally, intrauterine-produced stretch, although not proven to be sufficient to exceed the elastic limit of fetal peripheral nerve on its own [21,63,72], when coupled with externally-applied traction and various degrees of fetal head malpositioning (eg, asynclitism) or fetal acidosis, contributes to brachial plexus injury. There can thus be overlap between externally-applied traction that will or will not produce brachial plexus injury during shoulder dystocia, such that the difference in the degree of traction needed to produce an injury would be imperceptible to the delivering clinician. Even though the standard of care requires the avoidance of excessive traction during a shoulder dystocia delivery [73–75], in such a circumstance in which the degree of traction may be judged to have been within range of what other reasonably prudent clinicians practicing under similar circumstances might have used, the clinician's conduct in effecting such a delivery that culminated in an injury he or she likely caused would still have been within the standard of care.

Despite the above confounding issues concerning whether a clinician could have knowingly exceeded the elastic threshold of fetal peripheral nerve, there is an undeniable correlation between the extent of injury and the direction, magnitude, and rate of elongation (whether produced by uterine forces or clinician-applied forces) required to produce specific injury patterns [50,64,76,77]. In that sense, the severity of a resultant brachial plexus injury following shoulder dystocia, and not the permanence of the injury per se, does speak for itself in that it allows inference of the type and degree of externally-applied traction that more likely than not would have caused it.

Nevertheless, it is still not automatic that in every instance in which clinician-applied traction must have been outside the range of that usually used in difficult or shoulder-dystocia deliveries the degree of traction was below the standard of care. Once again, the specific clinical circumstances of the delivery must be considered. Just as may have been the case when a clinician chose to allow a trial of labor despite risk factors for shoulder dystocia, mitigating factors in the actual delivery may again present the clinician with the unenviable but necessary choice between two potential untoward outcomes, neither of which may be avoidable. If, despite the careful and competent efforts of the delivering clinician to resolve the shoulder dystocia, the head-to-body interval extends well outside the typical range for most shoulder dystocia (eg, beyond 6 to 8 minutes' duration), the risk for permanent central nervous system sequelae from asphyxia insult begins to override concerns over damaging the brachial plexus [17]. A standard-of-care–based argument can then be made that the use of a moderate to stout level of traction to ensure delivery in this circumstance was justifiable and consistent with reasonably prudent practice. The same argument can be proffered when the threat of asphyxial injury is accelerated by complete interruption of blood flow to the fetus, such as in the rare cases of coincident uterine rupture, complete placental abruption, or the need to clamp and cut the umbilical cord before delivery of the shoulders. In these circumstances, the same imperative for expeditious delivery by whatever means possible manifests much earlier in the head-to-body interval.

Counterarguments by defense

By this point in the article, the potential arguments that could be made in defense of the clinician being sued for his or her role in a shoulder dystocia–associated permanent brachial plexus injury should have become apparent to the reader; the gist of most of the above discussions concerning the fallacies of plaintiffs' allegations do form the basis for the standard shoulder dystocia defense strategy. Unfortunately, many defense lawyers (and their experts) can become as dogmatically monolithic and absolute in their approach as we have shown plaintiffs' counsel to be. The same sort of blurred distinctions between retrospective and prospective data that betray the validity of plaintiffs' absolutist arguments also diminish the plausibility of certain defense counterarguments. Much of defense attorneys' and their experts' evidence that shoulder dystocia and brachial plexus injury are incompletely linked or that injury cannot be prevented can be challenged by pointing out differences in shoulder dystocia definition and the failure to distinguish between causes of temporary as opposed to permanent injury [16]. Although plaintiffs try to conflate standard of care and causation leaving themselves vulnerable to the appearance of having unrealistic expectations of modern medicine and of its practitioners, defendants often are unwilling to yield on either standard of care or causation for fear that admitting the clinician's actions contributed the injury (even if it was entirely defensible) is necessarily perceived in the jurors' minds as a breach of the standard of care. Unfortunately, this uncompromising position can be imprudent, especially when the scientific foundation for other causes is significantly shaky. What follows is an analysis of the development and pitfalls of standard defense counterarguments in shoulder dystocia–associated brachial plexus injury.

Injury preceded physician involvement: uterine forces and shoulder dystocia itself cause the injury

Much of the recent obstetric literature on shoulder dystocia has focused on the claim that untoward outcomes are not the fault of the obstetric provider. The first efforts to support this theory involved an attempt to unlink the occurrence of brachial plexus injury from shoulder dystocia, thereby obviating the notion that clinician-applied traction would have been anything greater than routine and therefore the injury could not possibly bear any relationship to delivery technique. This thinking began with Jennett and colleagues [30] who discovered that half of newborn brachial plexus injuries were not associated with shoulder dystocia. Subsequently, a case report by Hankins and Clark [78] hypothesized that a permanent injury to the posterior arm in a litigated shoulder dystocia delivery could not have been the product of clinician-applied traction. Next, Ouzounian and colleagues reviewed 63 permanent brachial plexus injuries and concluded that there was no consistent obstetric risk factor among them [55].

All the non–shoulder dystocia injuries in Jennett et al's dataset were temporary, however, and therefore were not clinically or legally relevant [30]. In the case of the injury to the posterior arm, Hankins and Clark [78] had not been the treating physicians with first-hand knowledge of the delivery events or technique. Early obstetric texts illustrate upward flexion of the head and neck as a routine method for delivering the posterior shoulder. Allen and colleagues [67] discovered that in simulated shoulder-dystocia deliveries, when downward traction fails to deliver the anterior shoulder, the clinician frequently and consistently switches to upward traction (of similar magnitude to the original downward traction) in an attempt to deliver the posterior shoulder. Furthermore, the only prospectively documented spontaneous injury to the posterior arm reported by a treating clinician resolved by the fourth day of life, and although clearly not caused by the clinician, the injury was temporary and likely occurred by a mechanism substantially different from the cause of permanent brachial plexus injury [54]. It is undeniable that the preponderance of evidence suggesting a commonness of spontaneous brachial plexus injury following normal delivery or cesarean section is actually only relevant to temporary and not to permanent injury.

The attempt to separate brachial plexus injury from shoulder dystocia also suffers from failure to acknowledge differences between studies in shoulder dystocia reporting or definition. Although Ouzounian and colleagues [55] were unable to find differences in obstetric antecedents between injured and uninjured infants, 59 of the 63 permanent injuries had been shoulder-dystocia deliveries and the average birth weight among the 4 purportedly spontaneously injured children was greater than 4,000 g [79], which at least raises some suspicion that shoulder dystocia might not have been recognized in those cases or else might not have been documented in the record [80].

In their review, Gherman and colleagues [81] concluded that spontaneous delivery was a risk factor for permanent brachial plexus injury. Their rate of non–shoulder dystocia–related permanent birth injury was 1:1,000, the highest reported rate for permanent brachial plexus injury by a factor of seven [59]. This finding is likely the result of the authors having defined permanent injury as residual injury up to 1 year of age and their required use of ancillary maneuvers to accomplish delivery as the definition of shoulder dystocia, without regard to documentation of shoulder dystocia by the delivering clinician or documented head-to-body interval. We have found that clinicians diagnose a shoulder dystocia without the use of additional maneuvers beyond traction and episiotomy in 18% of deliveries in which there was difficulty in shoulder delivery [21]. Spong and colleagues [82] proposed an objective definition of shoulder dystocia, separate from the need for ancillary delivery maneuvers, as being met when the head-to-body interval exceeds 60 seconds. This theory was subsequently evaluated prospectively and determined to occur in one in seven deliveries [83], suggesting that obstructed delivery of the trunk occurs more commonly than previously believed, yet not infrequently goes underreported or unrecognized [84].

The first demonstrated case of legitimate permanent brachial plexus injury was a fatal one, caused by a neglected shoulder presentation [49]. Since then, the one compelling support for the alternative possibility of predelivery in utero pathogenesis for permanent brachial plexus injury was a report in 1980 by Koenigsberger [85] that documented two cases with electromyographic evidence of muscle denervation in infants less than 10 days old, which argued that Wallerian degeneration would have taken longer than 10 days to develop. The denervation injury therefore could not have coincided with the time of birth. This theory was subsequently debunked in an animal study by Gonik and colleagues [86] that demonstrated rapid development of Wallerian degeneration in neonatal peripheral nerve compared with adult nerve. Nevertheless, the spontaneous injury theory was in vogue until 2000, when Gonik and colleagues [87] suggested that the shoulder dystocia phenomenon itself (ie, the impaction of the shoulder behind the pubic symphysis coupled with intrauterine forces continuing to attempt expulsion of the fetus) may be responsible for the injury. They claimed incorrectly that uterine forces varied between 90 and 200 lbs, compared with only 22 lbs of clinician-applied traction, and that resultant brachial plexus stretch produced by endogenous forces was four to nine times higher than those produced by exogenous forces [87,88]. Besides there having been engineering principles that were violated in the initial model that had calculated uterine forces at 200 lbs, even the subsequently adjusted calculation of 90 lbs of uterine force remains three to four times greater than any intrauterine forces that have been measured clinically [72,89,90]. Most recently, the degree of stretch that occurs in utero before placement of traction on the fetal head has been shown experimentally to be well beneath the elastic threshold of fetal peripheral nerve [63]. In light of the preceding discussion, it becomes difficult to sustain a nonconciliatory stance on the issue of causation without appearing hopelessly unrealistic or to be suffering from self-serving denial. To these authors, the defense is more likely to present itself in a favorable light if instead they were to focus on an unwavering conviction that the standard of care was continually upheld, and that even so, the injury was caused by the actions of the clinician but was unavoidable.

Minimum necessary traction

A word of caution is needed concerning the claim that a permanent bra-chial plexus injury that occurred during shoulder dystocia was necessarily unavoidable. Lerner [91] puts forth a strategy that aims to shift the interpre-tation of the degree of traction that admittedly caused the injury from its having been excessive to its having been the minimum necessary to effect de-livery in an emergent situation. This characterization of traction is only rea-sonable when management of shoulder dystocia has been with appropriately executed maneuvers without persistence with a single, ineffective, traction-based maneuver (eg, McRoberts' maneuver or suprapubic pressure). It is important that the clinician progressed through other maneuvers of the shoulder dystocia management algorithm quickly to avoid the risk for injury [16,92].

A more critical determinant of brachial plexus injury during shoulder dystocia is the avoidance of increased magnitude, rate, or off-axis (in either the downward or upward direction) application of delivery traction force following each maneuver. Contrary to Lerner's argument, it is possible to generate enough force to resolve a shoulder dystocia by applying strong downward traction to the fetal head in a rapid, jerky, or torsional fashion, either before or after the use of shoulder dystocia maneuvers [50,51,76]. The severity of the dystocia may be such that hastily executed maneuvers, although sufficient to accomplish delivery, could also be accompanied by traction forces of a magnitude, direction, or rate that would be beyond the minimum necessary for that delivery.

Time is of the essence: the competing issue of asphyxial insult

One dominant belief concerning shoulder dystocia management is that the time window in which to resolve a shoulder dystocia before asphyxial insult would likely ensue is about 4 minutes. This belief is based on a math-ematically calculated decline in cord pH by 0.14 units per minute during the head-to-body interval [93]. None of 22 deliveries from which this time frame was extrapolated retrospectively had been complicated by shoulder dystocia or had sustained a head-to-body interval greater than 90 seconds' duration, however. Recent evidence suggests a much slower decline during shoulder dystocia deliveries [82,83,94], even among those associated with permanent brachial plexus injury [17]. We have previously reported on more than 200 severe shoulder dystocia deliveries in which no permanent CNS sequelae were incurred before 8 minutes' head-to-body interval, and after that initial 8-minute interval the decline in pH from the overall average pH of 7.24 did not reach statistical significance in either the injured or uninjured group [16]. The risk for hypoxic ischemic brain injury from asphyxia during shoulder dystocia thus does not have the linear relationship with time on the peri-neum as Wood originally suggested.

In contrast, the risk for brachial plexus injury from shoulder dystocia seems to increase continuously over the time, particularly when repeated attempts at traction on the fetal head with or without accompanying ancillary maneuvers, such as McRoberts' positioning, application of suprapubic pressure, and episiotomy, prove unsuccessful in accomplishing delivery. The force applied by the delivering clinician during repeated traction attempts is, more often than not, greater in magnitude than that applied during earlier attempts [51,67–69,95,96].

In the same severe shoulder-dystocia deliveries analyzed above, execution of fewer than two maneuvers per minute on the perineum was associated with increased risk for permanent brachial plexopathy [16,92]. Before an expert witness for the defense is able to justify the occurrence of a brachial plexus injury as unavoidable because it was preferable to the alternative of hypoxic ischemic encephalopathy as a long-term adverse outcome, there must be evidence of either a prolonged head-to-body interval in the face of unsuccessful yet multiple shoulder dystocia maneuvers or else some other mitigating circumstance that considerably shortens the 6- to 8-minute window available to likely resolve shoulder dystocia without asphyxial injury.

Proposed solutions to litigation crisis

There is no question that the current litigation crisis in obstetrics has alarming public health ramifications, including critical physician shortages in several areas of the United States caused by abandonment of obstetric practice as a result of prohibitive malpractice insurance premiums and improper use of medical resources and excessive health care spending spawned by defensive medical practices. Irrepressible propensity toward litigation in this country also impacts medical education, limiting the direct, hands-on training in skills needed to manage complicated or emergent medical conditions. Paradoxically, the threat of litigation has given rise to an appropriate heightened demand for patient safety standards but has simultaneously slowed the momentum for subjecting present-day shoulder dystocia management, which has significant limitations [21], to further critical analyses and scientific evaluation. The authors would contend that the most detrimental impact of the current litigation crisis is the impedance of the proper evolution of scientific inquiry needed to advance our knowledge of best practices, which should inform the development and refinement of present-day standards of care.

In response to the current crisis, many politicians and activist groups, both lay and professional, have proposed several solutions or reformations of the current tort system that is the domain of malpractice litigation. Although the efforts may have honorable intent, some of these proposed solutions, particularly as applied to shoulder dystocia–associated birth injury, have critical shortcomings that would either render them ineffective or would violate essential protective principles of United States civil law. These proposals and their limitations are addressed next. Again, we approach our critique from the viewpoint of academicians and not lawyers, concentrating on the fidelity and compatibility of proposed solutions to the medical circumstances surrounding shoulder dystocia–associated birth injury.

No-fault compensation programs

One intriguing proposition for tort reform is the establishment of a no-fault–type system of insurance and compensation for medical malpractice, akin to the paradigm of motor vehicle accident insurance and compensation plans. Rather than expecting perfect outcomes from birth, there would be the inherent expectation that accidents happen, often despite best intentions and proper actions of health care practitioners. Rather than attempting to sort out who is at fault, the victim should be entitled to compensation (at a preset level rather than left to be determined by individual jury panels) and should be guaranteed to receive such compensation based on the degree of injury and impairment suffered. Such a program is currently in effect in the state of Florida [97], and other states have considered adopting it also. The Florida plan is specifically for cerebral palsy; however, its potential applicability to other untoward outcomes from delivery has been proposed, including shoulder dystocia–associated Erb's palsy [98].

Setting aside legal, political, and economic analyses of whether such no-fault programs are successful in reducing litigation while effectively compensating affected individuals, there are important pathophysiologic (ie, injury mechanistic) differences between cerebral palsy and brachial plexus injury to consider that from a standpoint of applicability make a no-fault approach more difficult to use for the latter type of birth injury than for the former. First, most cerebral palsy–inducing asphyxial insults occur antenatally rather than intrapartum; nearly all permanent brachial plexus palsies are sustained during the birth process and do not predate the onset of labor.

Second, most antenatal causes for hypoxic ischemic encephalopathy (the precursor of cerebral palsy) escape clinical detection before birth or defy clinical intervention. Furthermore, the rare intrapartum antecedents of cerebral palsy, although detectable and potentially amenable to intervention, most often are sudden and catastrophic with nearly instantaneous effect, such that timely intervention is all but impossible even in the most ideal of clinical circumstances. Although shoulder dystocia most often occurs without warning, most incidents resolve atraumatically, and of those that do not, most incur only temporary injury, of which nearly all types (skeletal fractures, neurapraxias, or even third- and fourth-degree perineal lacerations) never require postdelivery treatment or compensation of any kind. Among those shoulder dystocias that result in permanent brachial plexus injury, however, the long-term outcome (ie, residual deficit) from such an injury is most often affected by the specific clinical management of the shoulder dystocia itself and by postnatal follow-up and treatment of the injury, both of which can be highly variable.

Finally, the deficit in cerebral palsy is, by definition, static and nonprogressive, such that its extent and expected natural history are more readily identifiable early in life and although the deficits can be managed and ameliorated with consistent clinical follow-up and therapeutic interventions there is little to offer in the way of repair. By contrast, most brachial plexus injuries, even if destined to have permanent sequelae, improve significantly over time. Unless severe, as in the rare cases involving the avulsion of nerve roots from the spinal cord, even those cases that seem to involve the entire plexus at birth show a typical centripetal recovery pattern up to 2 years postnatally. Furthermore, until there is (if there ever is) surgical exploration of the damaged brachial plexus with intraoperative neurophysiologic testing to characterize the extent of the damage and its effect on nerve conduction and muscle contraction patterns, most methods of nonoperative evaluation (including neuroimaging and electromyography) demonstrate limited and inconsistent long-term prognostic capability [99,100]. The outcome of permanent injury is also determined by the specificity, variety, and consistency of pediatric management [101]. Given that the relationship to the birth process, the role of the delivering clinician, and the pediatric follow-up, and the ability to prognosticate about long-term permanent sequelae soon after delivery are critical determinants of legitimate claims of medical malpractice and of limits to compensation for different types of birth injury, it seems doubtful that a system of no-fault compensation that would be not only applicable but also feasibly practicable for cerebral palsy would transfer easily to a birth injury, such as brachial plexus injury, that is so dissimilar in pathophysiology and prognosis.

Peer review of expert testimony

Another strategy for controlling malpractice litigation that has been gaining momentum in recent years is the proposed peer review of expert testimony. Concern has been raised over imbalances in the level of actual expertise between plaintiff and defense experts [102]. Even more fundamental is the unease over questionable veracity (from the point of view of medical plausibility) and consistency (within and between cases) of a given expert's testimony [103]. In theory, if experts' qualifications and the content of their opinions could be validated by a community of peers (ie, similar experts in the field) who would substantiate and differentiate the strength of medical evidence behind the statements made and ensure consistency of opinions proffered by confirming the similarity (or lack thereof) between the medical details of different cases in which such testimony is provided, then justice would be better served because court members would be more assured of the generalizability of the facts on which these cases are argued and decided.

The court system itself already has some methods and requirements in place for this type of control of expert testimony, such as the requirement for peer review and determination of merit before allowing malpractice litigation to be filed, the upholding of motions in limine, and the requirement (in federal jurisdictions) for substantiation of opinions through specific attribution to medical literature. Indeed, the privileges of discovery and cross-examination of witnesses afforded to counsel for both sides have been instituted to achieve some of these same ends. The general intent of many of the proponents of peer review is to effectively "police our own" mainly outside the court system—that is, to invoke the possibility of professional consequences (eg, loss of hospital privileges, revocation of membership in professional societies, or dismissal from academic departments) for the expert witness whose testimony is found wanting by the panel of peer professionals reviewing it. The hoped-for effect is that fewer experts would be willing to make dogmatic statements that fuel the absolutist arguments discussed above. This in turn would curb the level of compensation in those cases won by plaintiffs and with it the incentive to pursue litigation in the first place.

Although the authors would also be in favor of subjecting expert testimony to peer review on the same theoretic grounds given above, there are several considerations that warrant caution in how the academic obstetric community would proceed in such an effort. First, and most important, such reviews must be impartial and equally applied to plaintiff and defense experts with much the same objectivity and tenor we have attempted to set in this review. Careful assessment of the manner and source from which such peer review would be sought, and protection of mechanisms (internal and external) by which the expert witness retains recourse for disputing the determinations of the panel, are critical to avoiding accusations of abuse, impropriety, bias, or unfairness. Because there may be considerable differences between cases that are tried and those that never make it to a courtroom, and there are differences between jurisdictions in the possibility of pretrial examination of expert witnesses' opinions that thereby become a matter of public record, it is critical that the review panel considers the full breadth of cases in which a given expert has weighed in on standard of care and causation issues and has chosen to or has been given the opportunity (even after they have agreed) to support the side that requested their review. It is also important to maintain professional separation from interference in a legal system that, although beset by many imperfections and despite complex inadequacies related to other sources of inequality in our society, remains, in its constructs and precepts, among the best in the free world.

Until such matters are worked out in the proper channels and until permanent brachial plexus injury from shoulder dystocia is reduced as much as possible through optimization of current best practices on a wider, more generalizable scale, we continue to offer the following alternative approaches to litigation of shoulder dystocia–associated permanent brachial plexus:

- Maintenance of honesty and realistic expectations with patients: Acknowledging the difficulty of the delivery and of prognostication about the expected recovery from injury may help avert litigation in the first place.
- Documentation of pre-existing risks for shoulder dystocia and the planned mode of delivery as discussed with the patient: An honest appraisal of the lack of prospective evidence by which to realistically predict or avert shoulder dystocia and a discussion of the potential risks to alternative approaches are vital to the informed consent process.
- Education and familiarization of all providers with the indicated pediatric treatment and follow-up of injury: Parents should be encouraged to take a proactive approach to the ongoing evaluation and treatment of birth-related brachial plexus injury.
- Uncoupling of causation and standard of care during litigation: The decision to litigate a case and the strategy for defending the clinician's actions should be consistent with the most plausible explanations for pathogenesis without equating a clinician's role in producing the injury with necessarily breaching the standard of care.

References

[1] Mavroforou A, Koumantakis E, Michalodimitrakis E. Physicians' liability in obstetric and gynecology practice. Med Law 2005;24:1–9.
[2] Gilbert WM, Fadjo DE, Bills DJ, et al. Teaching malpractice for perinatal medicine and law. Obstet Gynecol 2003;101:589–93.
[3] Chauhan SP, Magann EF, McAninch CB, et al. Application of learning theory to obstetric maloccurence. J Matern Fetal Neonatal Med 2003;13:203–7.
[4] Geutjens G, Gilbert A, Helsen K. Obstetric brachial plexus palsy associated with breech delivery—a different pattern of injury. J Bone Joint Surg Br 1996;78:303–6.
[5] Hankins GDV, Speer M. Defining the pathogenesis and pathophysiology of neonatal encephalopathy and cerebral palsy. Obstet Gynecol 2003;102:628–36.
[6] O'Boyle AL, Davis GD, Calhoun BC. Informed consent and birth: protecting the pelvic floor and ourselves. Am J Obstet Gynecol 2002;187:981–3.
[7] Localio AR, Lawthers AG, Brennan TA, et al. Relation between malpractice claims and adverse events due to negligence: results of the Harvard medical practice study III. N Engl J Med 1991;325:245–51.
[8] Moore PJ, Adler NE, Robertson PA. Medical malpractice: the effect of doctor-patient relations on medical patient perceptions and malpractice intentions. West J Med 2000;173:244–50.
[9] Bellew M, Kay SP. Early parental experiences of obstetric brachial plexus palsy. J Hand Surg Br 2003;28:339–46.
[10] Hickson GB, Clayton EW, Githens PB, et al. Factors that prompted families to file medical malpractice claims following perinatal injuries. JAMA 1992;267:1359–63.
[11] Queenan JT. Professional liability–some solutions. Obstet Gynecol 2001;98:365–8.
[12] Simpson KR, Knox GE. Common areas of litigation related to care during labor and birth Recommendations to promote patient safety and decrease risk exposure. J Perinat Neonatal Nurs 2003;17:110–25.

[13] Kraman SS, Hamm G. Risk management: extreme honesty may be the best policy. Ann Intern Med 1999;131:963–7.

[14] Knox GE, Simpson KR, Garite TJ. High reliability perinatal units: an approach to the prevention of patient injury and medical malpractice claims. J Healthc Risk Manag 1999;19(2):24–31.

[15] Gurewitsch E, Kim E, Yang JH, et al. Comparing McRoberts' and Rubin's maneuvers for initial management of shoulder dystocia: an objective evaluation. Am J Obstet Gynecol 2005;192:153–60.

[16] Gurewitsch ED, Allen RH. Fetal manipulation for management of shoulder dystocia. Fetal and Maternal Medicine Review 2006;17:239–80.

[17] Allen RH, Rosenbaum TC, Ghidini A, et al. Correlating head-to-body delivery intervals with neonatal depression in vaginal births that result in permanent brachial plexus injury. Am J Obstet Gynecol 2002;187:839–42.

[18] Poggi SH, Stallings SP, Ghidini A, et al. Intrapartum risk factors for permanent brachial plexus injury. Am J Obstet Gynecol 2003;189:725–9.

[19] Poggi SH, Ghidini A, Allen RH, et al. Effect of operative vaginal delivery on the outcome of permanent brachial plexus injury. J Reprod Med 2003;48:692–6.

[20] Gurewitsch ED, Donithan M, Stallings S, et al. Episiotomy versus fetal manipulation in managing severe shoulder dystocia: a comparison of outcomes. Am J Obstet Gynecol 2004;191:911–6.

[21] Gurewitsch ED, Johnson E, Hamzehzadeh S, et al. Risk factors for brachial plexus injury with and without shoulder dystocia. Am J Obstet Gynecol 2006;194:486–92.

[22] Acker DB, Sachs BP, Friedman EA. Risk factors for shoulder dystocia. Obstet Gynecol 1985;66:762–8.

[23] Acker DB, Gregory KD, Sachs BP, et al. Risk factors for Erb-Duchenne palsy. Obstet Gynecol 1988;71:389–92.

[24] Acker DB, Sachs BP, Friedman EA. Risk factors for shoulder dystocia in the average-weight infant. Obstet Gynecol 1986;67:614–8.

[25] Allen RH, Poggi S, Stallings S, et al. Abnormality in the second stage of labor: a predictor of permanent brachial plexus injury due to shoulder dystocia. Am J Obstet Gynecol 2002;187:S169.

[26] Hassan AA. Shoulder dystocia: risk factors and prevention. Aust N Z J Obstet Gynaecol 1988;28:107–9.

[27] Geary M. Risk factors and fetal outcome in cases of shoulder dystocia compared with normal deliveries of a similar birthweight [letter]. Br J Obstet Gynaecol 1997;104:121–2.

[28] Benedetti TJ, Gabbe SG. Shoulder dystocia—a complication of fetal macrosomia and prolonged second stage of labor with midpelvic delivery. Obstet Gynecol 1978;52:526–9.

[29] Gonik B, Hollyer VL, Allen R. Shoulder dystocia recognition: differences in neonatal risks for injury. Am J Perinatol 1991;8:31–4.

[30] Jennett RJ, Tarby T, Kreinick CJ. Brachial plexus palsy: an old problem revisited. Am J Obstet Gynecol 1992;166:1673–7.

[31] Nesbitt T, Gilbert W, Herrchen B. Shoulder dystocia and associated risk factors with macrosomic infants born in California. Am J Obstet Gynecol 1998;179:476–80.

[32] Gilbert WM, Nesbitt TS, Danielsen B. Associated factors in 1611 cases of brachial plexus injury. Obstet Gynecol 1999;99:536–40.

[33] Sandmire HF, O'Halloin TJ. Shoulder dystocia: its incidence and associated risk factors. Int J Gynaecol Obstet 1988;26:65–73.

[34] Rouse DJ, Owen J, Goldenberg RL, et al. The effectiveness and costs of elective cesarean delivery for fetal macrosomia diagnosed by ultrasound. J Am Med Assoc 1996;276:1480–6.

[35] Phelan JP. Can we anticipate shoulder dystocia? Contemporary OB/GYN 1991;36:62–82.

[36] Donnelly V, Foran A, Murphy J, et al. Neonatal brachial plexus palsy: an unpredictable injury. Am J Obstet Gynecol 2002;187:1209–12.

[37] Sokol RJ, Blackwell SC. ACOG practice bulletin: shoulder dystocia. Number 40, 2002. Int J Gynaecol Obstet 2003;80:87–92.

[38] Mollberg M, Hagberg H, Bager B, et al. High birthweight and shoulder dystocia: the strongest risk factors for obstetrical brachial plexus palsy in a Swedish population-based study. Acta Obstet Gynecol Scand 2005;84:654–9.

[39] Iffy L. Common intrapartum denominators of shoulder dystocia related birth injuries. Zentralbl Gynakol 1994;116:33–7.

[40] Gonen O, Rosen DJ, Dolfinn Z, et al. Induction of labor versus expectant management in macrosomia: a randomized study. Obstet Gynecol 1997;89:913–7.

[41] Combs CA, Singh NB, Khoury JC. Elective induction versus spontaneous labor after sonographic diagnosis of fetal macrosomia. Obstet Gynecol 1993;81:491–6.

[42] Sanchez-Ramos L, Bernstein S, Kaunitz AM. Expectant management versus labor induction for suspected fetal macrosomia: a systematic review. Obstet Gynecol 2002;100: 997–1002.

[43] Bofill JA, Rust OA, Devidas M, et al. Shoulder dystocia and operative vaginal delivery. J Matern Fetal Med 1997;6:220–4.

[44] Towner D, Castro MA, Eby-Wilkens E, et al. Effect of mode of delivery in nulliparous women on neonatal intracranial injury. N Engl J Med 1999;341:1709–14.

[45] Murphy DJ, Liebling RE, Verity L, et al. Early maternal and neonatal morbidity associated with operative delivery in second stage of labour: a cohort study. Lancet 2001;358: 1203–7.

[46] Mollberg M, Hagberg H, Bager B, et al. Risk factors for obstetric brachial plexus palsy among neonates delivered by vacuum extraction. Obstet Gynecol 2005;106:913–8.

[47] Hankins GDV, Rowe TF. Operative vaginal delivery—year 2000. Am J Obstet Gynecol 1996;75:275–82.

[48] Poggi SH, Allen RH, Patel CR, et al. Randomized trial of McRoberts' versus lithotomy positioning to decrease the force that is applied to the fetus during delivery. Am J Obstet Gynecol 2004;191:874–8.

[49] Sever JW. Obstetric paralysis: its etiology, pathology, clinical aspects and treatment, with a report of four hundred and seventy cases. Am J Dis Child 1916;12:541–78.

[50] Baskett TF, Allen AC. Perinatal implications of shoulder dystocia. Obstet Gynecol 1995; 86:14–7.

[51] Allen RH, Sorab J, Gonik B. Risk factors for shoulder dystocia: an engineering study of clinician-applied forces. Obstet Gynecol 1991;77:352–5.

[52] Alfonso I, Dickson RA, Alfonso DT, et al. Fetal deformations: a risk factor for obstetrical brachial plexus palsy? Pediatr Neurol 2006;35:246–9.

[53] Graham E, Forouzan I, Morgan MA. A retrospective analysis of Erb's palsy cases and their relation to birth weight and trauma at delivery. J Matern Fetal Med 1997;6:1–5.

[54] Allen RH, Gurewitsch ED. Temporary Erb-Duchenne palsy without shoulder dystocia or traction to the fetal head. Obstet Gynecol 2005;105:1210–2.

[55] Ouzounian JG, Korst L, Phelan J. Permanent Erb's palsy: a lack of a relationship with obstetrical risk factors. Am J Perinatol 1998;15:221–3.

[56] Ubachs JMH, Slooff ACJ, Peeters LLH. Obstetric antecedents of surgically treated obstetric brachial-plexus injuries. Br J Obstet Gynaecol 1995;102:813–7.

[57] Ubachs JMH, Sloof ACJ. Aetiology. In: Gilbert A, editor. Brachial plexus injuries. London: Martin Dunitz; 2001. p. 151–7.

[58] Wolf H, Hoeksma AF, Oei SL, et al. Obstetric brachial plexus injury: Risk factors related to recovery. Eur J Obstet Gynecol Reprod Biol 2000;88:133–8.

[59] Morrison JC, Sanders JR, Magann EF, et al. The diagnosis and management of dystocia of the shoulder. Surg Gynecol Obstet 1992;175:515–22.

[60] Waters PM. Comparison of the natural history, the outcome of microsurgical repair, and the outcome of operative reconstruction in brachial plexus palsy. J Bone Joint Surg Am 1999;81:649–59.

[61] Sunderland S, Bradley KC. Stress-strain phenomena in human peripheral nerve trunks. Brain 1961;84:102–19.

[62] Alfonso I, Alfonso DT, Papazian O. Focal upper extremity neuropathy in neonates. Semin Pediatr Neurol 2000;7:4–14.

[63] Allen RH, Cha SL, Kranker LM, et al. Comparing mechanical fetal response during descent, crowning and restitution among deliveries with and without shoulder dystocia. Am J Obstet Gynecol, in press.

[64] Metaizeau JP, Gayet C, Plenat F. [Brachial plexus injuries: an experimental study]. Chir Pediator 1979;20:159–63 [in French].

[65] Slooff ACJ, Ubachs JMH. Brachial plexus impairment—a birth trauma? Am J Obstet Gynecol 1993;169:230.

[66] Gross SJ, Shime J, Farine D. Shoulder dystocia: predictors and outcome. Am J Obstet Gynecol 1987;156:334–6.

[67] Allen RH, Bankoski BR, Butzin CA, et al. Comparing clinician-applied loads for routine, difficult and shoulder dystocia deliveries. Am J Obstet Gynecol 1994;171:1621–7.

[68] Gonik B, Allen R, Sorab J. Objective evaluation of the shoulder dystocia phenomenon: effect of maternal pelvic orientation on force reduction. Obstet Gynecol 1989;74: 44–8.

[69] Crofts JF, Attilakos G, Read M, et al. Shoulder dystocia training using a new birth training mannequin. BJOG 2005;112:997–9.

[70] Tam W, Hoe YS, Huang S, et al. Measuring hand-applied forces during vaginal delivery without instrumenting the fetus or interfering with grasping function. J Soc Gynecol Investig 2004;11:S205A.

[71] Uysal II, Seker M, Karabulut AK, et al. Brachial plexus variations in human fetuses. Neurosurgery 2003;53:676–84.

[72] Buhimschi CS, Buhimschi IA, Malinow A, et al. Use of McRoberts' position during delivery and increase in pushing efficiency. Lancet 2001;358:470–1.

[73] Peleg D, Powell S. Shoulder dystocia: prediction, prevention, management, and defense. Postgraduate obstetrics and gynecology 1998;18:1–6.

[74] Dildy GA, Clark SL. Shoulder dystocia: risk identification. Clin Obstet Gynecol 2000;43: 265–82.

[75] Gross TL, Sokol RJ, Williams T, et al. Shoulder dystocia: a fetal-physician risk. Am J Obstet Gynecol 1987;15:1408–14.

[76] Morris WIC. Shoulder dystocia. J Obstet Gynaecol Br Emp 1955;62:302–6.

[77] Thorburn W. Obstetrical paralysis. J Obstet Gynecol 1903;3:454–8.

[78] Hankins GDV, Clark SL. Brachial plexus palsy involving the posterior shoulder at spontaneous vaginal delivery 1650. Am J Perinatol 1995;12:44–5.

[79] Ouzounian JG, Korst L, Phelan JP. Permanent Erb palsy—a traction-related injury? Obstet Gynecol 1997;89:139–41.

[80] Acker DB. Permanent Erb's palsy: a traction related injury [letter]. Obstet Gynecol 1997; 89:797.

[81] Gherman RB, Ouzounian JG, Miller D, et al. Spontaneous vaginal delivery-a risk factor for Erb's palsy? Am J Obstet Gynecol 1998;178:423–7.

[82] Spong CY, Beall M, Rodrigues D, et al. An objective definition of shoulder dystocia: prolonged head to body delivery intervals and/ or the use of ancillary obstetric maneuvers. Obstet Gynecol 1995;86:433–40.

[83] Beall MH, Spong C, McKay J, et al. Objective definition of shoulder dystocia: a prospective evaluation. Am J Obstet Gynecol 1998;179:934–7.

[84] Cohen AW, Otto SR. Obstetric clavicular fractures: a three-year analysis. J Reprod Med 1980;25:119–22.

[85] Koenigsberger MR. Brachial plexus palsy at birth: intrauterine or due to delivery trauma? Ann Neurol 1980;8:228.

[86] Gonik B, McCormick EM, Verwij BH, et al. The timing of congenital brachial plexus injury: a study of electromyography findings in the newborn piglet. Am J Obstet Gynecol 1998;178:688–95.

[87] Gonik B, Walker A, Grimm M. Mathematical modeling of forces associated with shoulder dystocia: a comparison of endogenous and exogenous sources. Am J Obstet Gynecol 2000; 182:689–91.

[88] Gonik B, Zhang N, Grimm MJ. Prediction of brachial plexus stretching during shoulder dystocia using a computer simulation model. Am J Obstet Gynecol 2003;189:1168–72.

[89] Reynolds SRM, Harris JS, Kaiser IH. Clinical measurement of uterine forces in pregnancy and labor. Springfield (IL): Charles C. Thomas; 1954. p. 124–43.

[90] Gonik B, Zhang N, Grimm MJ. Defining forces that are associated with shoulder dystocia: the use of a mathematic dynamic computer model. Am J Obstet Gynecol 2003;188:1068–72.

[91] Lerner H. Brachial plexus injury: the role of shoulder dystocia. Female Patient 2005;30: 12–6.

[92] Gurewitsch E, Stallings S, Tam W, et al. Does maneuver rate affect shoulder dystocia outcome? Am J Obstet Gynecol 2004;191:S66.

[93] Wood C, Ng KH, Hounslow D. Time—an important variable in normal delivery. J Obstet Gynaecol Br Commonw 1973;80:295–300.

[94] Stallings SP, Edwards RK, Johnson JWC. Correlation of head-to-body delivery intervals in shoulder dystocia and umbilical artery acidosis. Am J Obstet Gynecol 2001;185:268–74.

[95] Allen RH, Bankoski BR, Nagey DA. Simulating birth to investigate clinician-applied loads on newborns. Med Eng Phys 1995;17:380–4.

[96] Gurewitsch E, Cha S, Johnson T, et al. Traction training for routine and shoulder dystocia delivers: an experimental study. Am J Obstet Gynecol 2005;193:S41.

[97] Studdert DM, Fritz LA, Brennan TA. The jury is still in: Florida's birth-related neurological injury compensation plan after a decade. J Health Polit Policy Law 2000;25:499–526.

[98] Skolbekken JA. Shoulder dystocia—malpractice or acceptable risk? Acta Obstet Gynecol Scand 2000;79:750–6.

[99] Medina LS, Yaylali I, Zurakowski D, et al. Diagnostic performance of MRI and MR myelography in infants with a brachial plexus birth injury. Pediatr Radiol 2006;36:1296–9.

[100] Pitt M, Vredeveld JW. The role of electromyography in the management of obstetric brachial plexus palsies. Suppl Clin Neurophysiol 2004;57:272–9.

[101] Belzberg AJ, Dorsi MJ, Storm PB, et al. Surgical repair of brachial plexus injury: a multinational survey of experienced peripheral nerve surgeons. Neurosurg Focus 2004;16:1–11.

[102] Kesselheim AS, Studdert DM. Characteristics of physicians who frequently act as expert witnesses in neurologic birth injury litigation. Obstet Gynecol 2006;108:273–9.

[103] Hammond CB, Schwartz PA. Ethical issues related to medical expert testimony. Obstet Gynecol 2005;106:1055–8.

CLINICS IN
PERINATOLOGY

Clin Perinatol 34 (2007) 387–392

Group B Streptococcus Infection in Pregnancy

Hung N. Winn, MD, JD, MBA

Department of Obstetrics, Gynecology and Women's Health, University of Missouri-Columbia School of Medicine, 3401 Berrywood, Suite 203, Columbia, MO 65201, USA

Group B streptococcus (GBS) (*streptococcus agalactiae*), a gram-positive coccus, is one of the major causes of maternal or neonatal severe infection and sepsis. Maternal infection associated with GBS includes acute chorioamnionitis, endometritis, and urinary tract infection. Neonatal GBS infection is characterized as early onset if occurring within 7 days of age or late onset otherwise, and involves bacteremia, pneumonia, or meningitis [1,2].

Epidemiology

Five percent to 40% of all pregnant women in the United States have rectovaginal colonization with GBS [3–5]. In patients who have preterm labor or preterm premature rupture of membranes, the incidence of genital colonization of GBS is 15% [6]. One percent to 5% of urinary tract infections result from GBS colonization [7]. The incidence of neonatal GBS infection is 1.8 per 1000 live births [7]. Neonatal colonization of GBS may occur as a result of in utero ascending infection from the maternal genital tract or direct contact during delivery. Vertical transmission from the mother to the neonate by either method accounts for up to 75% of cases of neonatal GBS colonization, and 1% to 2% of these infants will develop early-onset GBS infection [9–13]. The case fatality of early-onset GBS neonatal infection varies from 11% to almost 50% [8,14–16]. Maternal risk factors that predispose a neonate to early-onset GBS infection include preterm delivery, prolonged rupture of membranes (> 18 hours), intrapartum fever temperature of at least 38° C or 100.4° F, or prior infant who had GBS infection [17]. The risk of neonatal GBS colonization from a GBS colonized mother is 45.5 per 1000 live births if maternal fever, prolonged rupture of

E-mail address: winnh@health.missouri.edu

membranes, and preterm birth coexist [18]. Late-onset GBS neonatal infection may occur from maternal–neonatal transmission, or nosocomial or community contacts [19,20].

Diagnosis

Group B streptococcal colonization can be detected by either culture or rapid diagnostic tests. Currently, culture remains the gold standard of diagnosing GBS colonization [17]. The yield of positive GBS culture is increased by sampling the anorectum in addition to the vagina because the gastrointestinal tract is a major reservoir of GBS [5,21,22]. This can be done in a single swab. Inhibition of competing organism by using a selective medium such as Todd-Hewitt broth, which contains gentamicin, polymyxin B, and validixic acid, also increases the yield of the GBS culture [1]. The main limitation of culture is time. Because culture results are not available for 24 to 48 hours, management may be problematic if delivery is imminent.

Rapid-diagnostic tests of GBS directly detect the extracted specific polysaccharide antigen. The available tests use either latex particle agglutinization or enzyme immunoassay. These tests are easy to perform, are generally less expensive than a culture, and produce results within a short period of time (usually within 1 hour). Although rapid-detection tests are highly sensitive in patients who are heavily colonized with GBS, their overall rates of sensitivity and high false-negative results compared with those of cultures prevent their widespread clinical application [23–27]. These drawbacks for the rapid diagnostic tests also exist in the setting of preterm labor or preterm premature rupture of membranes demonstrates that the rapid latex agglutination fails to identify GBS neonatal infection in one heavily, two moderately, and three lightly colonized mothers. More importantly, the overall sensitivity of the latex agglutination test in identifying maternal–neonatal pairs at risk for GBS neonatal infection is only 25% [6].

Treatment

Intrapartum chemoprophylaxis is effective in reducing the attack rate of early-onset neonatal GBS [18]. The American College of Obstetricians and Gynecologists recommends screening pregnant women at 35 to 37 weeks and provides intrapartum chemoprophylaxis for those who have positive cultures for rectovaginal GBS colonization [17]. Currently, prenatal treatment of colonized pregnant patients with oral antibiotics is not recommended because this approach unlikely eradicates maternal genial GBS colonization at the time of labor and delivery. Thirty percent to 70% of pregnant patients who received antenatal ampicillin or aqueous penicillin for genital colonization of GBS remain colonized at delivery [28,29].

The use of antibiotics in preventing early-onset neonatal GBS infection in the settings of preterm delivery premature rupture of membranes with prolonged latent phase remains to be determined. One approach is to initiate antibiotic treatment pending genital culture result. If the culture is negative, the antibiotic is discontinued; otherwise the antibiotic is continued orally for a week. The genital GBS cultures are repeated weekly to determine the additional course of chemoprophylaxis. The patient should receive intrapartum chemoprophylaxis if she ever had genital GBS colonization during her pregnancy regardless of the results of intervening GBS cultures and/or treatments.

Intrapartum chemoprophylaxis

Aqueous penicillin G (PCN G) is the drug of choice with the initial dose of 5 million units intravenously and maintenance dose of 2.5 million units intravenously every 4 hours. Ampicillin is the alternative with the initial dosage of 2 g and the maintenance dose of 1 g every 4 hours. Penicillin G is preferable to ampicillin because of its narrower spectrum of bacterial sensitivity, thus less likely causing the selective emergence of other pathogenic bacterias [17,30]. Because the bactericidal level in the maternal serum can obtained with a dose of 1 million units of PCN G IV every 4 hours, the lower dose may be sufficient [31]. Furthermore, maternal administration of ampicillin or penicillin should be attempted despite imminent delivery, because bactericidal levels of penicillin or ampicillin in the maternal or fetal blood can be reached within 5 minutes of maternal administration of ampicillin or penicillin, respectively [31–33]. In addition, there is no significant correlation between maternal body mass index and maternal or fetal serum levels of ampicillin [33]. Women who have a history of PCN allergy but are at low risk for PCN anaphylaxis should receive cefazolin instead of clindamycin or erythromycin [30] because of the increasing resistance of GBS to these antibiotics [34,35]. Cefazolin can be given with the initial dose of 2 g IV and a maintenance dose of 1 g intravenously every 8 hours [17,30]. The mean concentration of cefazolin that inhibits 90% of GBS isolates (MIC_{90}) is rapidly reached in the maternal serum, amniotic fluid, and fetal serum after maternal administration of cefazolin [36]. Women who are at high risk for PCN anaphylaxis should receive either (1) clindamycin 900 mg every 8 hours or erythromycin 500 mg every 6 hours if GBS is susceptible to clindamycin or erythromycin, or (2) vancomycin 1 g intravenously every 12 hours if GBS is resistant to both clindamycin and erythromycin or GBS susceptibility to these two antibiotics is unknown. Currently, group B streptococcus is 100% susceptibility to PCN G, ampicillin, and vancomycin. However, only 91% and 79% of GBS isolates are susceptible to clindamycin and erythromycin, respectively [35]. Intrapartum chemoprophylaxis should be given intravenously until delivery.

Legal consideration

A care provider would be liable to the patients if he/she breaches the standard of care owed to the patients who subsequently sustain injury.

Although the standard of care may vary with the clinical situation, the approach as discussed in this article would provide guidelines for developing the individual standard of care. Clinicians should be aware of the following pitfalls that may lead to suboptimal care: (1) improper collection of specimen for GBS culture due to poor technique or incorrect timing; (2) untimely availability of GBS culture results, especially when the specimen is sent to the outside laboratory; (3) preterm delivery or premature rupture of membranes before 35 weeks of gestation due to either maternal or fetal indications; and (4) improper administration of chemotherapy due to delay or selection of the ineffective antibiotics. The hospital may want to develop a system to have such medications as PCN G and ampicillin available on the labor and delivery unit so that the medication can be promptly administered. It is important to recognize that care providers incur liability to the patients only if the deviation from the standard of care causes the neonatal injury as a result of GBS infection. Adverse neonatal outcomes could be due to maternal or fetal conditions that are unrelated to maternal or neonatal GBS colonization.

Summary

Although controversy exists regarding screening and treatments, there is a consensus that chemoprophylaxis in the intrapartum period dramatically reduces the rate of infection in the mother and neonate. At present, the most effective strategy of reducing early-onset GBS infection is antenatal maternal screening for rectovaginal GBS colonization at 35 to 37 weeks of gestation and intrapartum treatment of patients who have: (1) positive maternal GBS screening, (2) positive GBS urine culture during the current pregnancy, and (3) a previous infant who had GBS infection. Penicillin G is the drug of choice for this purpose, and ampicillin is the alternative. Cefazolin may be used in patients who have a low risk for PCN allergy, whereas clindamycin or vancomycin can be used in those at high risk for PCN allergy. Maternal vaccination, being developed, seems to be the most cost-effective measure in preventing early onset GBS neonatal infection.

References

[1] Baker CJ. Summary of the workshop on perinatal infections due to group B streptococcus. J Infect Dis 1977;136:137–52.
[2] Faro S. Group B beta-hemolytic streptococci and puerperal infections. Am J Obstet Gynecol 1981;139:686–9.
[3] Anthony BF, Okada DM, Hobel CJ. Epidemiology of group B streptococcus: longitudinal observations during pregnancy. J Infect Dis 1978;137:524–30.
[4] Regan JA, Klebanoff MA, Nugent RP. Vaginal Infections and Prematurity Study Group. The epidemiology of group B streptococcal colonization in pregnancy. Obstet Gynecol 1991;77:604–10.

[5] Dillon HC, Gray E, Pass MA, et al. Anorectal and vaginal carriage of group B streptococci during pregnancy. J Infect Dis 1982;145:794–9.

[6] Winn HN, McLennan M, Amon E. Clinical assessment of the rapid latex agglutination screening test for group B streptococcus. Int J Gynecol Obstet 1994;47:289–90.

[7] Schwartz B, Schuchat A, Oxtoby MJ, et al. Invasive group B streptococcal disease in adults: a population-based study in metropolitan Atlanta. JAMA 1991;266:1112–4.

[8] Zangwill KM, Schuchat A, Wenger JD. Group B streptococcal disease in the United States, 1990: report from a multistate active surveillance system. In: CDC Surveillance Summaries. MMWR Morb Mortal Wkly Rep 1992;41(No. SS-6):25–32 (November 20, 1992).

[9] Jones DE, Kanarek KS, Lim DV. Group B streptococcal colonization patterns in mothers and their infants. J Clin Microbiol 1984;20:438–40.

[10] Francois RA, Knostman JD, Zimmerman RA. Group B streptococcal neonate and infant infections. J Pediatr 1973;82:707.

[11] Hood M, Janney A, Dameron G. Betahemolytic streptococcus group B associated with problems of the perinatal period. Am J Obstet Gynecol 1961;82:809.

[12] Baker CJ, Barrett FF. Transmission of group B streptococci among parturient women and their neonates. J Pediatr 1973;83(6):919–25.

[13] Baker CJ, Edwards MS. Group B streptococcus infections: perinatal impact and prevention methods. Ann NY Acad Sci 1988;549:193–202.

[14] Schuchat A, Oxtoby M, Cochi S, et al. Population-based risk factors for neonatal group B streptococcal disease: results of a cohort study in metropolitan Atlanta. J Infect Dis 1990; 102:672–7.

[15] Dars MA, Gray BM, Khare S, et al. Prospective studies of group B streptococcal infections in infants. J Pediatr 1979;95:437–43.

[16] Opal SM, Cors A, Palmer M, et al. Group B streptococcal sepsis in adults and infants. Arch Intern Med 1988;148:641–5.

[17] American College of Obstetricians and Gynecologists. Prevention of early-onset group B streptococcal disease in newborns. ACOG Comm Opin 2002;279:1405–12.

[18] Boyer KM, Gotoff SP. Prevention of early onset neonatal group B streptococcal disease with selective intrapartum chemoprophylaxis. N Engl J Med 1986;314:1665–9.

[19] Yow MD, Leeds LJ, Mason EO, et al. The natural history of group B streptococcal colonization in the pregnant woman and her offspring. I. Colonization studies. Am J Obstet Gynecol 1980;137:34–8.

[20] Anthony BF, Okada DM, Hobel CJ. Epidemiology of the group B streptococcus: maternal and nosocomial sources for the infant acquisitions. J Pediatr 1979;95:431–6.

[21] Badri MS, Zawaneh S, Cruz AC, et al. Rectal colonization with group B streptococcus: relation to vaginal colonization of pregnant women. J Infect Dis 1977;135:308–12.

[22] Philipson EH, Palermino DA, Robinson A. Enhanced antenatal detection of group B streptococcus colonization. Obstet Gynecol 1995;85:437–9.

[23] Kontrick C, Edberg S. Direct detection of group B streptococci from vaginal specimens compared with quantitative culture. J Clin Microbiol 1987;25:573–4.

[24] Wald E, Dashefsky B. Rapid detection of group B streptococci directly from vaginal swabs. J Clin Microbiol 1987;25:573–4.

[25] Skoll MA, Mercer BM. Evaluation of two rapid group B streptococcal antigen tests in labor and delivery patients. Obstet Gynecol 1991;77:322–6.

[26] Gentry YM, Hillier SL. Evaluation of two rapid enzyme immunoassay for detection of group B streptococcus. Obstet Gynecol 1991;78:397–401.

[27] Granab PA, Petosa MT. Evaluation of a rapid screening test for detecting group B streptococci in pregnant women. J Clin Microbiol 1991;29:1536–8.

[28] Hall RT, Barnes W, Krishnan L, et al. Antibiotic treatment of parturient women colonized with group B streptococci. Am J Obstet Gynecol 1976;124:630–4.

[29] Gardner SE, Yow MD, Leeds LJ, et al. Failure of penicillin to eradicate group B streptococcal colonization in the pregnant woman: a couple study. Am J Obstet Gynecol 1979;135:1062–5.

[30] Centers for Disease Control and Prevention. Prevention of perinatal group B streptococcal disease: revised guidelines from CDC. MMWR Morb Mortal Wkly Rep 2002;51(No. RR-11).

[31] Johnson JR, Colombo DF, Gardner D, et al. Optimal dosing of penicillin G in the third trimester of pregnancy for prophylaxis against group B streptococcus. Am J Obstet Gynecol 2001;185(4):851–3.

[32] Bloom SL, Cox SM, Bawdon RE, et al. Ampicillin for neonatal group B streptococcal prophylaxis: how rapidly can bactericidal concentrations be achieved? Am J Obstet Gynecol 1996;175:974–6.

[33] Colombo DF, Lew JL, Pedersen CA, et al. Optimal timing of ampicillin administration to pregnant women for establishing bactericidal levels in the prophylaxis of group B streptococcus. Am J Obstet Gynecol 2006;194:466–70.

[34] Pearlman MD, Pierson CL, Faix RG. Frequent resistance of clinical group B streptococci isolates to clindamycin and erythromycin. Obstet Gynecol 1998;92:258–61.

[35] Edwards RK, Clark P, Duff P, et al. Intrapartum antibiotic prophylaxis 2: positive predictive value of antenatal group B streptococci cultures and antibiotic susceptibility of clinical isolates. Obstet Gynecol 2002;100(3):540–4.

[36] Mitchell TF, Pearlman MD, Chapman RL, et al. Maternal and transplacental pharmacokinetics of cefazolin. Obstet Gynecol 2001;98(6):1075–9.

The Placenta as Witness

Rebecca N. Baergen, MD

New York Presbyterian Hospital, Weill-Cornell Medical Center,
Department of Pathology, Starr 1002, 520 East 70th Street,
New York, NY 10021, USA

In 1991, the American College of Obstetrics and Gynecology published a practice bulletin [1], broadly stating, "The benefit of securing specimens on a routine basis is as yet unproved, a standard approach to placental pathology cannot be recommended." The expression of this opinion was unfortunate, because it perpetuated a misconception about the importance of placental pathology despite evidence to the contrary and at the same time discouraged even cursory examination of the placenta. It is true that most placentas, like most infants, are normal. However, when an infant is injured or abnormal in some way, numerous studies have shown that the placenta plays an instrumental role in ascertaining the cause of the adverse outcome and in the defense of obstetricians and other health care workers when there are allegations of malpractice [2]. Fortunately, there has recently been increased interest in the placenta in medicolegal cases, where the placenta has played a pivotal role, and at times, stood in the forefront, not only as participant but also as witness.

One of the most common reasons for litigation is unexpected adverse outcome, in particular cerebral palsy and various types of neurologic injury, neurologic impairment, or developmental delays. Cerebral palsy is a group of nonprogressive neurodevelopmental disorders recognized in early childhood [3], typically characterized by abnormalities in movement and posture but also involving abnormalities in sensation, cognition, communication, perception, and behavior. There seems to be no uniform cause, and thus the possible etiologies have been debated for many years. While some authors opine that 90% of the cases of cerebral palsy are not due to intrapartum events [4], other authors have countered by stating that most are due to problems in the perinatal period [5]. Unfortunately, this controversy is

E-mail address: rbaergen@med.cornell.edu

unlikely to be resolved in the near future. Nevertheless, placental examination has much to offer in the understanding of adverse perinatal outcome.

The placenta is the most important fetal organ because it is responsible for exchange of all nutrients, oxygen, and fluid from mother to fetus and removal of fetal waste products. It has also been called the "diary of gestational life" [6]—an extremely appropriate description. The placenta not only reflects the intrauterine environment, but also can provide valuable information on the cause and timing of many adverse events and conditions. This includes neurologic injury and many other fetal conditions, such as fetal distress, infections, growth restriction, and demise, as well as identification of unsuspected maternal disorders, such as lupus or maternal vascular disease, and primary placental disorders, such as maternal floor infarction or chronic villitis. Furthermore, the placenta, being a fetal organ, expresses the fetal genotype and thus may provide diagnostic information on various genetic, chromosomal, congenital, or hematologic disorders.

In the context of adverse outcome, examination of the placenta may be helpful in several ways. First, the placenta may be the cause of the adverse outcome due to an inherent abnormality, such as maternal floor infarction, or a primary placental lesion, such as an umbilical cord knot or a massive chorangioma. Second, adverse outcome may be due to disease processes that are not placental in origin but that lead to abnormal placental function such as maternal underperfusion and fetal thrombotic vasculopathy. In other situations, the placenta is functioning normally but reflects an abnormal intrauterine environment or an adaptation to adverse conditions such as chorangiosis or increased nucleated red blood cells. Finally, the placenta may be normal, in which case certain conditions may be ruled out and thus one's attention is directed elsewhere to look for the cause of injury. Not only may the etiology of the injury be ascertained from placental examination, but also a time frame during which the abnormal condition has been operating. Acute lesions may be associated with sudden catastrophic events whereas other, more chronic, lesions develop over a period of time leading to decreased placental reserves at a minimum (Table 1). Markedly depleted reserves will render the infant susceptible to stresses of labor and to more acute events and therefore may also be associated with significant injury or death.

Acute placental processes

Acute processes involving the placenta are usually the result of an acute interruption of maternal or fetal blood flow. These are usually either due to traumatic events, mechanical obstruction, or disruption and may be associated with acute fetal blood loss. Interruption of maternal blood may be caused by uterine rupture or separation of the placenta from the uterus (placental abruption), whereas interruption of fetal blood flow will result from disruption or obstruction of fetal vessels in the placenta (see Table 1).

Table 1
Categories of placental pathology

Type of lesion	Acute placental processes	Chronic placental processes
Affecting maternal blood supply	Uterine rupture Acute placental abruption	Maternal underperfusion Chronic placental abruption Infarction/ischemic change Villous morphologic change Accelerated villous maturity Increased syncytial knots Decidual vasculopathy
Affecting fetal blood supply	Acute obstruction of blood flow Umbilical cord occlusion Acute fetal hemorrhage Disruption of large fetal vessels Velamentous vessels Disruption of fetal capillaries Fetomaternal hemorrhage Fetal trauma	Partial or chronic obstruction of blood flow Umbilical cord occlusion Fetal thrombotic vasculopathy Meconium associated myonecrosis
Primary placental lesions		Maternal floor infarction Chronic villitis Meconium associated myonecrosis
Inflammatory/Infectious processes		Acute chorioamnionitis With fetal inflammatory response With fetal thrombosis Chronic villitis
Abnormal intrauterine environment		Nucleated red blood cells Chorangiosis

Disruption of blood flow to the uterus from traumatic uterine rupture due to a motor vehicle accident, previous cesarean section, or other trauma may lead to sudden, severe fetal hypoxia sufficient to cause severe neurologic injury or death [7]. If uterine rupture leads to life-threatening hemorrhage necessitating hysterectomy, pathologic examination of the uterus will reveal the rupture and demonstrate dissection of blood into the uterine wall. Acute abruption, in which the placenta acutely separates from the uterus before delivery of the infant, will cause complete loss of blood flow to the placental tissue underlying the abruption. An acute abruption of 50% of the placenta will lead to fetal death [8], and lesser separations and those occurring less acutely can lead to sublethal injury [2,9,10]. If cesarean section is performed, direct visualization of the placental detachment is possible, while pathologic examination of the placenta will show a retroplacental clot, often with compression of underlying villous tissue (Fig. 1). If an infant is delivered within an hour or so of placental separation, the retroplacental clot will not be tightly adherent to the basal plate, and thus confirmation of the abruption

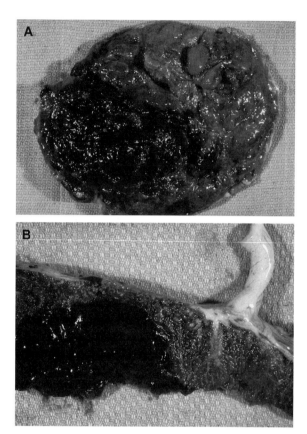

Fig. 1. Acute abruption. (*A*) Maternal surface of the placenta with fresh retroplacental clot
(*left*) covering approximately 50% of the surface. (*B*) Cut surface of same placenta showing
compression of villous tissue underneath retroplacental hematoma. *From* Baergen RN. Manual
of Benirschke and Kaufmann's Pathology of the Human Placenta. New York, NY: Springer;
2005; with kind permission of Springer Science and Business Media.

cannot be made. However, within a few hours, early changes occur including the presence of a recent retroplacental clot with dissection of blood
through the decidua and villous stromal hemorrhage. Over the next few
hours, the clot begins to indent the villous tissue, and there are progressive
indications of ischemic change in the underlying chorionic villi with villous
agglutination and eventually infarction [11]. Over a period of many days,
the infarction eventually becomes a firm tan-white scar. Thus, based on extent and progression of the villous damage, the timing of the abruption can
be estimated. However, even acute abruptions often do not develop all at
once but rather extend over time, complicating interpretation.

As the umbilical cord is the lifeline of the fetus, obstruction or disruption
of blood flow through the umbilical vessels is capable of leading to severe

fetal compromise. Most types of obstruction are mechanical in nature and are associated with compression of the umbilical cord. Acute obstruction of blood flow through the fetal circulation may be caused by cord entanglement, tight true knots, excessively twisted or constricted cords, compression of membranous vessels, or cord prolapse. If obstruction is complete and does not resolve, fetal or neonatal death will be the result [2,12–17]. Obstruction may also be partial or complete, but complete obstruction, even for a short time, is likely to lead to neurologic damage. This is supported by studies showing that long cords, excessively twisted cords, constrictions and velamentous insertion are significantly more common in infants who have cerebral palsy [9,12,18]. In any type of cord compression, the umbilical vein, being more distensible than the arteries, will be compressed initially and solely in more minor types of compression. Thus, venous return of oxygenated blood from the placenta to the fetus will be diminished, resulting in venous and capillary congestion in the placenta and, often, a certain degree of hypovolemia and anemia in the fetus. In acute compression, histologic sections of the placenta will show distension of the umbilical vessels, particularly the vein; tributaries of the umbilical vein in the chorionic plate; and villous capillaries. These findings are nonspecific and thus do not enable the definitive diagnosis of cord compression as the cause of cerebral palsy in a specific case. Direct compression of a portion of the cord by fetal parts or the cervix may also cause "bruising" of the cord with nonspecific damage or degenerative change of Wharton's jelly and the umbilical vessels.

Disruption of fetal vessels will result in acute fetal hemorrhage, which can result in severe hypovolemia and circulatory collapse. Hemorrhage may result from disruption of fetal vessels anywhere in the vascular tree, from the large umbilical vessels all the way down to the small villous capillaries [16]. Disruption of larger vessels will result in a large fetal hemorrhage quickly, whereas hemorrhage from small vessels tends to be more chronic but may still be significant. The most common origin of large vessel hemorrhage is disruption of velamentous vessels. Velamentous vessels are present in velamentous and furcate insertions of the umbilical cord, between accessory lobes and occasionally in marginal cord insertions. Without the protection of Wharton's jelly, these membranous vessels are susceptible to damage, particularly after membrane rupture when the added protection afforded by the amniotic fluid is lost. In vasa previa, velamentous vessels cross the cervical os, preceding the presenting fetal part and are especially susceptible to damage. Examination of the placenta is essential to document the presence of velamentous vessels as well as the disruption of those vessels and the hemorrhage into the surrounding tissues (Fig. 2). It is essential that the suspicion of ruptured velamentous vessels be communicated to the pathologist before examination so that extra care can be taken to preserve the pathologic findings. Rarely, rupture of the umbilical cord itself may occur if there is excessive traction due to a short cord [19], from abnormal adherence of the placenta due to placenta accreta, or from pathologic

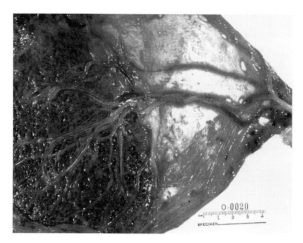

Fig. 2. Velamentous cord insertion with disruption. Disrupted velamentous vessels are seen at the right; fresh hemorrhage into the membranes is seen at far right and bottom of the figure. *From* Baergen RN. Manual of Benirschke and Kaufmann's Pathology of the Human Placenta. New York, NY: Springer; 2005; with kind permission of Springer Science and Business Media.

processes that make the cord more friable, such as necrotizing funisitis [20], ulceration due to meconium damage [21], aneurysms of umbilical vessels [11], hemangiomas [11], or trauma. Trauma may be inflicted from fetal blood sampling, direct trauma to the fetus, or amniocentesis [16]. With large vessel hemorrhage, significant blood loss can occur within mere minutes, often leading to fetal death or severe neurologic damage quickly. The etiologies of cord rupture are rare, and pathologic examination is necessary to document the specific underlying lesion in each case. However, placental findings generally indicative of severe fetal anemia are a markedly pale placental parenchyma (Fig. 3), a marked increase in nucleated red blood cells in fetal placental vessels, villous edema and intervillous thrombi.

A specific type of acute exsanguination may occur in monozygotic twins with monochorionic placentas. In these placentas, vascular anastomoses are always present to some degree. In some cases, there is a dominant artery to vein anastomosis, which results in a chronic shunt of blood from one twin, the donor, to the other twin, the recipient. This is the basis for the twin-to-twin transfusion syndrome. However, even when this syndrome is not present, there is always the potential for acute transfusion of blood from one twin to the other [16]. If one twin dies in utero, the dead twin, lacking a blood pressure, becomes a "sink" into which the surviving twin bleeds. Depending on the size of the anastomoses, hemorrhage can lead to various outcomes from minimal blood loss to profound neurologic injury or death, all of which will occur within a matter of minutes of fetal death of the cotwin [22]. The surviving twin will be severely anemic and the corresponding placenta will be markedly pale.

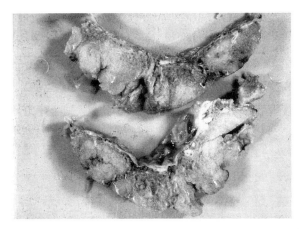

Fig. 3. Severe fetal hemorrhage. Cut section of placental parenchyma shows pale villous tissue indicative of severe fetal anemia. *From* Baergen RN. Manual of Benirschke and Kaufmann's Pathology of the Human Placenta. New York, NY: Springer; 2005; with kind permission of Springer Science and Business Media.

Fetal hemorrhage from the much smaller villous capillaries will cause fetal blood to escape into the intervillous space, resulting in a fetomaternal hemorrhage. In many cases of fetomaternal hemorrhage, there are multiple episodes leading to chronic blood loss. Placental findings include multiple or large intervillous thrombi and evidence of fetal anemia, but these are not readily identifiable in every case. Fetomaternal hemorrhage is thought to develop when there is damage to the trophoblastic covering of the villi [16], but in most cases, the exact cause is obscure and there is usually no history of trauma. Fetomaternal hemorrhage is seen with increased frequency in the presence of placental choriocarcinomas and large placental hemangiomas (chorangiomas) [23]. The diagnosis of this condition usually rests on identification of fetal blood in the maternal circulation, which is most commonly confirmed by the Kleihauer-Betke test, although other tests such as the Apt test or flow cytometry have also been used. The Kleihauer-Betke test is reported as a percentage of fetal blood cells in the maternal circulation, but there may be confounding factors. A falsely low result will be obtained if mother and infant are ABO incompatible, thus causing the fetal blood cells to be quickly cleared from her circulation, whereas maternal persistence of fetal hemoglobin will lead to a falsely elevated result. Generally, fetal cells persist in the maternal circulation for several weeks, so performing the test is useful even if it is done several days or more after delivery. It is strongly recommended that it be performed in any case in which neonatal anemia is diagnosed.

Chronic placental processes

Chronic placental lesions develop due to long-standing and ongoing conditions, over a period of days to weeks and result in a decrease in placental reserves. They consist of abnormalities in maternal blood supply, fetal blood supply, primary placental lesions, and inflammatory lesions, and most of these lesions are easily identifiable on pathologic examination (see Table 1). When chronic placental lesions are present in the setting of a small placenta, there is a decrease in the total surface area for oxygen and nutrient exchange, which may result in poor fetal growth. Thus, small placentas are often associated with small or growth-restricted infants. Growth restriction itself is a significant risk factor for cerebral palsy [24,25]. Even when chronic lesions are present in normal sized placentas, placental function is diminished due to damage to the placental parenchyma, and placental reserves are thus also diminished. Under normal conditions, one quarter to a third of the placenta may be damaged without a significant adverse affect on oxygen exchange. However, when chronic processes have resulted in a placenta with little or no reserves, the infant is particularly susceptible to additional insults that may occur during labor and delivery [25].

The most common condition in this category is maternal underperfusion in which abnormalities in the maternal circulation and maternal blood vessels lead to diminished uteroplacental perfusion [26]. Often "uteroplacental sufficiency" is used in this context, but this term is at best imprecise, and it is preferable to be specific about the placental lesion or abnormality. The most common clinical associations are hypertensive diseases including preeclampsia, eclampsia, and chronic hypertension, but systemic lupus erythematosus, anticardiolipin antibodies, and inherited coagulopathies have also been associated with lesions of malperfusion. In some cases, no underlying clinical condition is evident. Pathologically, the most diagnostic lesion is decidual vasculopathy, which consists of abnormalities in the decidual or uteroplacental vessels. These vessels show various alterations including fibrinoid necrosis, atherosis, mural hypertrophy, and lack of normal physiologic conversion [11,16,26]. The implication of these changes is twofold. First, there is the development of morphologic changes in the chorionic villi, which can be adaptive or maladaptive. Specifically, the villi may show an appearance of accelerated maturity with smaller size and increased syncytial knots, which increases surface area and oxygen exchange. In severe and long-standing malperfusion, the villi do not mature adequately and the terminal villi do not properly form, a form of hypoplasia, which is a clearly maladaptive response. Second, the chorionic villi undergo ischemic change. The earliest manifestation is villous agglutination with collapse of the intervillous space and adherence of adjacent villi to one another. No longer perfused by maternal blood in the intervillous space, they ultimately become infarcted. Decidual necrosis and bleeding from abnormal decidual vessels can lead to acute and chronic placental separation (abruption). If sufficient placental parenchyma is nonfunctional, there will be a critical point at which seemingly small acute stresses lead to catastrophic events. This is in contrast to milder forms of malperfusion in which there may be some adaptation to hypoxic conditions, and compensatory mechanisms may provide some protection against neurologic injury [9,10,27].

Decreased placental reserves also occur when there is chronic obstruction of blood flow in the fetal circulation due to thrombosis in the fetal circulation, or fetal thrombotic vasculopathy [13,28,29]. Chronic obstruction in the fetal circulation, like acute obstruction, is often related to mechanical forces exerted on the umbilical cord. Studies have shown that abnormally twisted cords, short cords, long cords, velamentous cord insertions, and cord constrictions are associated with an increased risk of fetal demise, neurologic injury, and abnormal developmental outcome [2,9,12–14,17–20] as has thrombosis of fetal placental vessels [28,29]. Except for cord entanglement, these lesions are easily diagnosed grossly on placental examination if the observer is familiar with normal cord parameters. Partial obstruction of blood flow through the cord leads to decreased venous return from the placenta, venous stasis, and subsequent thrombosis in the fetal circulation, which can further embarrass blood supply to the fetus. A hypercoaguable state in the fetus may also result in thrombosis [29]. These lesions can cause a significant loss of oxygen carrying capacity and placental reserves.

There are several thrombotic lesions comprising this group, some of which can be recognized grossly (Fig. 4) [28,30]. They include occlusive and nonocclusive thrombi, mural thrombi, intimal fibrin cushions, avascular villi, and hemorrhagic endovasculopathy (villous stromal–vascular karyorrhexis) [30]. Most commonly, the larger vessels in the chorionic plate and in the stem villi are affected. On microscopic examination, recent thrombi contain fibrin, clot, and extracellular material. Older thrombi are recognizable by the presence of calcification within the lumen or the wall of the vessel and indicate duration of many weeks. Lack of blood flow in the fetal circulation will eventually lead to involution of the "downstream" villi, resulting in the formation of avascular villi, a process also occurring over a period of

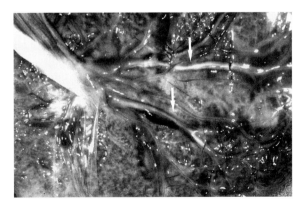

Fig. 4. Thrombosis of fetal chorionic vessels. Fetal surface of the placenta with arrows indicates grossly visible thrombi in fetal chorionic vessels. *From* Baergen RN. Manual of Benirschke and Kaufmann's Pathology of the Human Placenta. New York, NY: Springer; 2005; with kind permission of Springer Science and Business Media.

weeks. Avascular villi, as the name suggests, are chorionic villi containing somewhat hyalinzed stroma and no fetal vessels. Hemorrhagic endovascul-opathy, also called hemorrhagic endovasculosis or hemorrhagic endovascu-litis, is most commonly, but not exclusively, found in the smaller villous capillaries [31,32]. It is opined that obstruction of blood flow leads to dam-age of the vascular wall, necrosis, and extravasation of blood into the stroma. However, this lesion may be an intermediate lesion in the evolution of avascular villi, and thus the term villous stromal–vascular karyorrhexis has also been used [30]. Hemorrhagic endovasculopathy alone has been linked to adverse neurologic outcome [32,33].

Primary placental lesions

Primary placental lesions are a heterogeneous group with varied etiology; however, they all either interfere with maternal or fetal blood flow or lead to villous destruction. The lesions most pertinent to adverse outcome are ma-ternal floor infarction, chronic villitis, and meconium associated myonecro-sis. As they are chronic processes, they can significantly decrease placental reserves and thus have been associated with cerebral palsy, neurologic in-jury, or neonatal encephalopathy [9,25,28,32–35].

Maternal floor infarction, also called massive perivillous fibrin deposi-tion, is a lesion of unknown etiology characterized by a marked deposition of fibrin or fibrinoid in the intervillous space, with fibrinoid material coating the surfaces of the chorionic villi [11,16]. In its extreme form, most of the placental parenchyma is involved, and the oxygen and nutrient-carrying ca-pacity of the placenta is markedly diminished. Even though the villi are still viable at this point, being deprived of their blood supply, they will eventu-ally become completely infarcted. Maternal floor infarction is strongly asso-ciated with fetal growth restriction, and stillbirth [16,36,37] and studies have also shown a link with adverse long-term neurologic outcome [34]. The eti-ology is not completely clear, but it has been suggested that it is an immune-mediated response. This is supported by the common presence of fibrinoid at the maternal–fetal interface and its high rate of recurrence (up to 50%) in subsequent pregnancies [37].

Chronic villitis is defined as an infiltrate of chronic inflammatory cells in the chorionic villi. It may be of two types: infectious villitis and villitis of un-known etiology, the latter being the most common as it occurs to at least a mild degree in 5% of placentas [11,16]. Although illitis of unknown etio-logyis an inflammatory process, it is considered a primary placental lesion. Like maternal floor infarction, it is often present at the maternal–fetal inter-face and has a high recurrence rate [16]. The inflammatory cells have been shown to be primarily maternal in origin [38], and thus, like maternal floor infarction, is thought to represent a type of host versus graft response in which the mother "rejects" the placenta. It is characterized histologically by a lymphohistiocytic infiltrate in the chorionic villi and intervillous space.

It can occasionally be necrotizing with widespread villous destruction and then is associated with loss of continuity in the fetal circulation, vascular occlusion, and thrombosis. Severe diffuse chronic villitis is seen significantly more common in infants who have cerebral palsy and neurologic injury [9,28,39].

Meconium is the intestinal content of the fetus, and discharge of meconium into the amniotic fluid is a common event especially in term or post-term infants. It usually does not lead to significant problems. In a small percentage of cases, meconium is aspirated by the fetus, and then meconium aspiration syndrome may develop, which is associated with significant neonatal morbidity and mortality. Furthermore, meconium is a noxious material, containing bile salts, enzymes, and other compounds [8]. If meconium is present in the amniotic fluid for a sustained period, it will cause damage to the lining of the amniotic cavity, the umbilical cord, and fetal vessels. Initially, within a few hours of meconium exposure, there is a degenerative change of the amnionic epithelium of the fetal membranes and chorionic plate and pigment-filled macrophages become visible on microscopic examination [8,40]. After 12 to 16 hours or more, damage to the umbilical cord can take place [8]. The damage manifests as necrosis of the vascular smooth muscle of the umbilical vessels, most commonly the arteries, and is readily identified on histologic section. In addition, in vitro studies have shown that meconium causes vasoconstriction of umbilical vessels [21,35]. Vasoconstriction is more likely to occur in longer meconium exposure and when there is meconium associated myonecrosis. Because this will compromise blood flow, it is not unexpected that meconium associated myonecrosis is associated with a significant risk of neurologic injury and cerebral palsy [9,28].

Acute chorioamnionitis and fetal inflammatory response

Acute chorioamnionitis is defined histologically, as acute inflammatory cells within the fetal membranes, the amnion and the chorion. It is indicative of an ascending bacterial infection, an infection in the amniotic cavity. Initially, the inflammatory response to bacteria that enter the uterine cavity is maternal in origin. If the infection continues and goes unchecked, there will be a fetal inflammatory response with acute inflammatory cells migrating out of fetal vessels in the umbilical cord (acute funisitis) and chorionic plate. This can lead to subsequent damage to fetal blood vessels and fetal vascular thrombosis. These events generally occur over a period of days. If the fetus becomes infected, decreased pulmonary function and oxygenation may develop due to acute bronchopneumonia, and if the fetus becomes septic, systemic effects such as hypotension and decreased vascular perfusion will result. Ascending infection is a major cause of preterm labor and delivery, which is, by itself, a significant risk factor for cerebral palsy [16]. Even without fetal infection, exposure of the fetus to the bacteria will elicit a fetal inflammatory response with the production of cytokines and inflammatory mediators. In preterm infants, cytokines interfere with maturation of oligo-dendrocytes. In term and preterm infants, there are many systemic and central nervous system effects. In particular, the permeability of the blood brain barrier is altered and there are vasoactive effects leading to hypoperfusion of the brain and direct toxic effect on the brain by inflammatory mediators [9,28,41]. Thus, the presence of a severe fetal inflammatory response and associated thrombosis has been linked to adverse neurologic outcome, periventricular leukomalacia, and cerebral palsy in many studies [9,28,41–43].

Abnormal intrauterine environment

In some cases, placental examination does not point to a cause of neurologic injury or evidence of decreased placental reserves but reflects an attempt at adaptation to an abnormal and perhaps hostile intrauterine environment. There are two main placental findings in this category, nucleated red blood cells and chorangiosis, both of which are indicators of intrauterine hypoxia [16,43]. When hypoxia is present, the kidneys respond by producing erythropoietin, increasing the formation of red blood cells in fetal hematopoietic organs to increase the oxygen-carrying capacity of the blood. In so doing, immature nucleated red blood cells are put into the circulation prematurely. An increase in nucleated red blood cells in the fetal circulation will be seen on microscopic examination of the placenta and is an exact reflection of the fetal circulation at the time of delivery. The increase is more accurately measured in the first blood cell count on the neonate where a quantitative value can be ascertained. An absolute count greater than $2500/cm^3$ is considered indicative of significant hypoxia. The time it takes for this elevation to occur is somewhat controversial [9,16]. One of the reasons for this is that the fetus has stores of already formed nucleated red blood cells that it can release under hypoxic conditions. Therefore, a modest elevation may take place quickly, probably within an hour or less. In contrast, for a more marked increase, there must be time for additional red blood cell precursors to form, and therefore these increases take more time, likely at least 12 to 24 hours [6,8,44].

The second finding, chorangiosis, is also indicative of intrauterine hypoxia. Chorangiosis is an adaptive response on the part of the placenta wherein there is a proliferation of villous capillaries, presumably in an attempt to increase oxygen-carrying capacity. There are specific criteria used to establish this diagnosis [45,46], but often less stringent criteria are used. For chorangiosis to develop, the hypoxia must be of sufficient magnitude and duration to provide adequate stimulus for the creation of new blood vessels, a process that takes weeks. As with nucleated red blood cells, the underlying cause may be obscure. Chorangiosis has been associated with adverse perinatal and neonatal outcomes such as neonatal death, low Apgar scores, and admissions to the neonatal ICU [45].

Summary

Placental lesions associated with adverse neurologic outcome can be divided into those with abnormal blood flow in the maternal circulation (maternal underperfusion), abnormal blood flow in the fetal circulation (primarily fetal thrombotic vasculopathy), inflammatory processes, and primary placental lesions. Each are associated with identifiable pathologic lesions. Neurologic injury can occur by way of sudden, acute, and possibly devastating events by way of ongoing chronic processes that primarily lead to decreased placental and fetal reserves, or by way of a combination of both. Generally speaking, pathologic examination provides more information on chronic as opposed to acute events, but this is largely dependent on the specific pathologic process one is studying, because many acute events can be diagnosed or confirmed on placental examination. In neurologically impaired infants, often multiple placental lesions are present and timing of all lesions present can provide a "storyline" of events in the development of an adverse intrauterine environment. Multiple lesions of different etiologies and involving different aspects of placental function (eg, fetal versus maternal blood circulation) can act synergistically to decrease placental reserves and function. The same is true when acute events occur in combination with chronic processes [9]. The presence of multiple placental lesions greatly increases the susceptibility of the fetus to neurologic injury, as recent studies have borne out [9,28,47].

The extent to which placental pathology can be helpful in understanding adverse antenatal and perinatal events varies with the type and significance of placental lesions. Interpretation of these lesions is complex and requires experience and insight into clinicopathologic correlation with outcome. Although ultimately this may require some expertise in placental pathology, the most important part of placental examination is ensuring that it is performed. In any case, where adverse outcome is suspected, the placenta should be secured for proper examination. It is highly recommended that, in addition, a photographic record be made of any potential gross pathologic findings. If there is adequate gross examination and submission of tissue, the information the placenta provides will be available for many years to come. The placenta alone may not provide the complete answer but is an important and essential witness in understanding adverse outcome.

References

[1] Committee on Obstetrics. Maternal and fetal medicine. ACOG committee opinion number 102. Placental pathology. December 1991. Int J Gynaecol Obstet 1992;39:146–7.
[2] Grafe MR. The correlation of prenatal brain damage with placental pathology. J Neuropathol Exp Neurol 1994;53(4):407–15.
[3] Bax M, Goldstein M, Rosenbaum P, et al. Proposed definition and classification of cerebral palsy. Dev Med Child Neurol 2005;47(8):571–6.
[4] Maclennan A. A template for defining a causal relation between acute intrapartum events and cerebral palsy: international consensus statement. BMJ 1999;319:1054–9.

[5] Cowan R, Rutherford M, Groenendaal F, et al. Origin and timing of brain lesions in term infants with neonatal encephalopathy. Lancet 2003;361(9359):736–42.
[6] Altshuler G. Some placental considerations in alleged obstetrical and neonatology malpractice. In: Wecht CH, editor. Legal medicine. Salem (NH): Butterworth Legal Publishers; 1994. p. 27–47.
[7] Phelan JP, Ahn MO, Korst L, et al. Intrapartum asphyxial brain injury with absent multiorgan system dysfunction. J Matern Fetal Med 1998;7(1):19–22.
[8] Benirschke K. The use of the placenta in the understanding of perinatal injury. In: Donn SM, Fisher CW, editors. Risk management techniques in perinatal and neonatal practice. Armonk (NY): Futura publishing Co, Inc.; 1996. p. 325–45.
[9] Redline RW, O'Riordan A. Placental lesions associated with cerebral palsy and neurologic impairment following term birth. Arch Pathol Lab Med 2000;124:1785–91.
[10] Baergen RN. Manual of Benirschke and Kaufmann's pathology of the human placenta. New York: Springer; 2005.
[11] Kumazaki Kaori, Nakayama M, Sumida Y, et al. Placental features in preterm infants with periventricular leukomalacia. Pediatr 2002;109(4):650–5.
[12] Machin GA, Ackerman J, Gilbert-Barnass E. Abnormal umbilical cord coiling is associated with adverse perinatal outcomes. Pediatr Dev Pathol 2000;3(5):462–71.
[13] Redline RW. Clinical and pathological umbilical cord abnormalities in fetal thrombotic vasculopathy. Hum Pathol 2004;35:1494–8.
[14] Peng HQ, Levitin-Smith M, Rochelson B, et al. Umbilical cord stricture and overcoiling are common causes of fetal demise. Pediatr Dev Pathol 2006;9(1):14–9.
[15] Murphy DJ, MacKenzie IZ. The mortality and morbidity associated with umbilical cord prolapse. Br J Obstet Gynaecol 1995;102(10):826–30.
[16] Benirschke K, Kaufmann P, Baergen RN. Pathology of the human placenta. Fifth edition. New York: Springer; 2006.
[17] Spellancy WN, Gravem H, Fisch RO. The umbilical cord complications of true knots, nuchal coils and cords around the body. A report from the collaborative study of cerebral palsy. Am J Obstet Gynecol 1966;94(8):1136–42.
[18] Baergen RN, Malicki D, Behling CA, et al. Morbidity, mortality and placental pathology in excessively long umbilical cords. Pediatr Dev Pathol 2001;4:144–53.
[19] Miller ME, Higginbottom M, Smith DW. Short umbilical cord: its origin and relevance. Pediatr 1981;67:618–21.
[20] Chasen ST, Baergen RN. Necrotizing funisitis with intrapartum umbilical cord rupture. J Perinatol 1999;19(4):325–6.
[21] Altshuler G, Arizawa M, Molnar-Nadasdy G. Meconium induced umbilical cord vascular necrosis and ulceration; a potential link between the placenta and poor pregnancy outcome. Obstet Gynecol 1992;79:760–6.
[22] Karsidag ATK, Kars B, Dansuk R, et al. Brain damage to the survivor within 30 minutes of co-twin demise in monochorionic twins. Fetal Diagn Ther 2005;20:91–5.
[23] Santamaria M, Benirschke K, Carpenter PM, et al. Transplacental hemorrhage associated with placental neoplasms. Pediatr Pathol 1987;7(5–6):601–15.
[24] Jarvis S, Glinianaia SV, Torrioli M, et al. Cerebral palsy and intrauterine growth in single births: European collaborative study. Lancet 2003;362:1106–11.
[25] Redline RW, Patterson P. Patterns of placental injury: correlations with gestational age, placental weight and clinical diagnosis. Arch Pathol Lab Med 1994;118:698–701.
[26] Redline RW, Boyd T, Campbell V, et al. Maternal vascular underperfusion: nosology and reproducibility of placental reaction patterns. Pediatr Dev Pathol 2004;7:237–9.
[27] Burke CJ, Tannenberg AE. Prenatal brain damage and placental infarction: an autopsy study. Dev Med Child Neurol 1995;37:555–62.
[28] Redline RW. Severe fetal placental vascular lesions in term infants with neurologic impairment. Am J Obstet Gynecol 2005;192:452–7.

[29] Kraus FT, Acheen VI. Fetal thrombotic vasculopathy in the placenta: cerebral thrombi and infarcts, coagulopathies and cerebral palsy. Hum Pathol 1999;30:759–69.

[30] Redline RW, Ariel I, Baergen RN, et al. Fetal vascular obstructive lesions: nosology and reproducibility of placental reaction patterns. Pediatr Dev Pathol 2004;7:443–52.

[31] Sander CH. Hemorrhagic endovasculitis and hemorrhagic villitis of the placenta. Arch Pathol Lab Med 1980;104:371–3.

[32] Sander CH, Kinnane L, Stevens NG. Hemorrhagic endovasculitis of the placenta: a clinico-pathologic entity associated with adverse pregnancy outcome. Compr Ther 1985;11:66–74.

[33] Sander CM, Gilliland D, Akers C, et al. Livebirths with placental hemorrhagic endovascu-litis: interlesional relationships and perinatal outcomes. Arch Pathol Lab Med 2002;126: 157–64.

[34] Adams-Chapman I, Vaucher YE, Bejar RF, et al. Maternal floor infarction of the placenta: association with central nervous system injury and adverse neurodevelopmental outcome. J Neonatol 2002;22:236–41.

[35] Altshuler G, Hyde S. Meconium-induced vasocontraction: a potential cause of cerebral and other fetal hypoperfusion and of poor pregnancy outcome. J Child Neurol 1989;4:137–42.

[36] Andres RL, Kuyper W, Resnik R, et al. The association of maternal floor infarction of the placenta with adverse perinatal outcome. Am J Obstet Gynecol 1990;163(3):935–8.

[37] Katzman PJ, Genest DR. Maternal floor infarction and massive perivillous fibrin deposi-tion: histological definitions, association with intrauterine growth restriction, and risk of recurrence. Pediatr Dev Pathol 2002;5(2):159–64.

[38] Redline RW, Patterson P. Villitis of unknown etiology is association with major infiltration of fetal tissues by maternal inflammatory cells. Am J Pathol 1993;143:473–9.

[39] Scher MS, Trucco GS, Beggarly ME, et al. Neonates with electrically confirmed seizures and possible placental associations. Pediatr Neurol 1998;19:37–41.

[40] Miller PW, Coen RW, Benirschke K. Dating the time interval from meconium passage to birth. Obstet Gynecol 1985;66:459–62.

[41] Bejar RF, Wozniak P, Allard M, et al. Antenatal origin of neurologic damage in newborn infants. I. Preterm infants. Am J Obstet Gynecol 1988;159(2):357–63.

[42] Redline RW, Wilson-Costello D, Borawski E, et al. The relationship between placental and other perinatal risk factors for neurologic impairment in very low birth weight children. Pediatr Res 2000;47(6):721–6.

[43] Hermansen MC. Nucleated red blood cells in the fetus and newborn. Arch Dis Child Fetal Neonatal Ed 2001;84:F211–5.

[44] Blackwell SC, Hallak M, Hotra JW, et al. Timing of fetal nucleated red blood cell count elevation in response to acute hypoxia. Biol Neonat 2004;85:217–20.

[45] Altshuler G. Chorangiosis: an important placental sign of neonatal morbidity and mortality. Arch Pathol Lab Med 1984;10:71–4.

[46] Soma H, Watanabe Y, Hata T. Chorangiosis and chorangioma in three cohorts of placentas from Nepal, Tibet and Japan. Reprod Fertil Dev 1996;7:1533–8.

[47] Viscardi RM, Sun CJ. Placental lesion multiplicity: risk factor for IUGR and neonatal cra-nial ultrasound abnormalities. Early Hum Dev 2001;62:1–10.

CLINICS IN
PERINATOLOGY

Clin Perinatol 34 (2007) 409–438

Causation—Fetal Brain Injury and Uterine Rupture

Jeffrey P. Phelan, MD, JD[a,*],
Lisa M. Korst, MD, PhD[b],
Gilbert I. Martin, MD[c]

[a]*Department of Obstetrics and Gynecology, Citrus Valley Medical Center, West Covina, CA, USA*
[b]*Department of Obstetrics and Gynecology, USC Keck School of Medicine, 12439 Magnolia Blvd., Suite 154, North Hollywood, CA 91607, USA*
[c]*University of California Irvine, Citrus Valley Medical Center, 1135 South Sunset Avenue, Suite 406, West Covina, CA 91790, USA*

Perinatal litigation is not a stranger to the practicing obstetrician. Whether the claim involves preeclampsia [1] or fetal brain injury [2,3], these lawsuits are, in general, more often related to the severity of the injury and the age of the patient [4] than they are related to matters of quality of care. In many cases the more severe the patient's injury and the younger the patient, the greater is the potential for a lawsuit to be filed and a subsequent settlement or award to be made. Because obstetricians typically provide care to young women and their fetuses, death or disability to the mother or her fetus that is attributable to any medical or obstetric condition has the potential to result in a large award or settlement. Unfortunately for the obstetrician or any provider of health care to a pregnant woman, the alleged obstetric malpractice is all too frequently linked to the severity of the injury and not to the quality of care rendered [4].

The concept of causation, or whether the provider contributed to or caused the resultant injury to a patient, is an integral part of the prosecution or the defense of any obstetric malpractice claim. Causation is the cornerstone or the nexus between the alleged breach in the standard of care and the patient's injury. It is also important to understand that as part of any causation analysis, the plaintiff's goal is to return the injured party to whole

* Corresponding author. 13181 Crossroads Parkway North, Suite 380, City of Industry, CA 91746.
    E-mail address: phelanjp@earthlink.net (J.P. Phelan).

0095-5108/07/$ - see front matter © 2007 Elsevier Inc. All rights reserved.
doi:10.1016/j.clp.2007.03.014   *perinatology.theclinics.com*

or to the status the person would have been had the person not been injured because of the alleged negligence of the obstetrician or the hospital personnel. Returning the patient to whole means that the patient is made economically, physically, and emotionally whole. This concept is not limited to physical injuries.

The purpose of this article is to familiarize the reader with the concept of causation in the setting of an obstetric malpractice case. To provide insights into this complicated area, the concept of foreseeability of harm is introduced along with its potential application in the daily practice of obstetrics and in obstetric malpractice law suits. These concepts are covered in several hypothetical fetal brain injury cases. This discussion involves an overview of available scientific evidence used to substantiate or refute whether a child's brain damage or maternal uterine rupture was, in fact, related to the obstetric care in question. For example, in a brain-damaged baby case, causation typically centers on whether the fetal brain injury arose intrapartum or at some other time outside the window of labor and delivery, and whether the fetal brain injury was potentially preventable. Although causation in a uterine rupture case is typically focused on the role of uterine stimulators and uterine activity patterns, the discussion explores available scientific evidence to determine if there is any support for those theories. In the event of the delivery of a depressed newborn, a checklist of scientific evidence to be gathered at the time of delivery is also provided. This article is directed toward obstetric providers, is intended to be used solely for educational purposes, and is not designed to provide legal advice. It is hoped that this article ultimately results in a greater understanding of the role of causation in an obstetric malpractice claim and the pathogenesis of fetal injuries and uterine rupture. It is anticipated that obstetric providers will be able to implement many of these concepts into their continued efforts to improve perinatal outcome.

Negligence and causation

To establish whether a defendant committed medical malpractice, the plaintiff must prove their case by a preponderance of the evidence, which means that the scales of justice only need to be tilted in favor of the plaintiff or the defendant. This condition requires that the plaintiff satisfy or the defense refute in some way the four elements of negligence. These four elements are duty, breach, causation, and injury. The plaintiff must demonstrate that the obstetrician had a duty or obligation to the patient and for some reason breached that duty to the patient. The alleged breach in the standard of care must then have contributed to or caused the patient's injury. The legal standard to prove causation is to a degree of medical probability or certainty. As demonstrated in Fig. 1, the element of causation serves as the nexus or bridge between the alleged breach in the standard

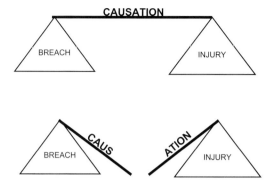

Fig. 1. Causation serves as the bridge or nexus between any alleged breach in the standard of care and the patient's resultant injuries.

of care and the resultant injury. If there is no causal link to the patient's injuries, or the bridge collapses, the plaintiff cannot show that the patient's injury was caused by or related to the breach in the standard of care. Theoretically, causation stands as a fortress against whether an obstetric malpractice claim survives.

Because causation can provide a reasonable explanation of what happened, matters of causation are often times readily understood by the jury. One of the key issues that relates to causation and its analysis by the trier of fact is that the scientific information is usually contained within the medical records. When the matter goes to the judge or jury, the medical records usually go into the jury room. It is thus important for the providers of obstetric care to gather as much evidence as possible surrounding an adverse outcome and make sure the information is documented in the medical records. This documentation includes written descriptions of the event and also any pertinent laboratory data on the mother or child. In the case of a depressed newborn, data collection is quintessential; this is covered in more detail elsewhere in this article.

Foreseeability of harm

The concept of foreseeability of harm, first coined by Justice Benjamin Cardozo in 1916, is firmly entrenched in our legal system and serves as a road map for any and all obstetric malpractice litigation. This concept, which is taught to every aspiring lawyer in America, has its roots in the case of MacPherson v Buick Motor Company [5]. In that case, Justice Cardozo wrote that "because the danger is to be foreseen, there is a duty to avoid the injury...if [a person] is negligent where a danger is to be foreseen, a liability will follow" [5].

The simplest example for the application of this legal principle is the typical stop sign case. Stop signs are positioned to protect drivers from the inherent dangers related to entering and proceeding through intersections. If, for example, two cars enter the intersection simultaneously, it is reasonably foreseeable that an accident could result. Stop signs thus impose an obligation or a duty on drivers who approach that intersection to stop before proceeding through it. If a driver fails to stop, it is reasonably foreseeable that the two cars could crash. The driver who runs the stop sign thus could be held liable for any resultant property damage or personal injuries. The application of this concept in the medical–legal setting demonstrates quickly the differences in the training of physicians and lawyers. Figs. 2 and 3 illustrate the differing perspectives of these two professionals with respect to a fetal heart rate (FHR) bradycardia. The obstetric providers in Fig. 2 reflexively respond by delivering the fetus in the most expeditious manner. The lawyer in Fig. 3, conversely, asks whether the obstetrician/nurse should have seen the FHR bradycardia coming and thus avoided the FHR bradycardia altogether. In other words, were the obstetric providers on notice of the pending bradycardia?

Notice

If an event is considered foreseeable or potentially avoidable (eg, the sudden appearance of repetitive severe variable FHR decelerations in a patient undergoing a vaginal birth after a cesarean [VBAC] followed by a FHR bradycardia), the obstetrician/nurse is considered to be on notice of a uterine rupture. Notice means the circumstances in which a physician or nurse has sufficient time to identify the potential for acute fetal distress and an ample opportunity to correct or prevent the problem through timely intervention or heightened scrutiny. The legal test thus becomes one based on "what a reasonably prudent obstetrician/nurse would foresee and would do in light of [that information] under the circumstances" [6] in this case, this time. Although the test imposes an affirmative obligation to act, it is also used to link the obstetric conduct to the outcome. The more foreseeable the fetal brain damage or uterine rupture is, the greater is the likelihood that the obstetric care provided will be causally linked to the fetal outcome.

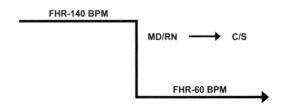

Fig. 2. The perspective of the physician and the nurse in the situation of fetal distress. BPM, beats per minute; MD, medical doctor; RN, registered nurse. (*Reproduced from* Phelan JP. Perinatal risk management: obstetric methods to prevent birth asphyxia. Clin Perinatol 2005;32: 1–17; with permission.)

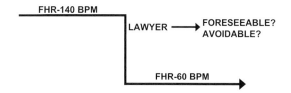

Fig. 3. The perspective of an attorney in the situation of fetal distress. BPM, beats per minute. (*Reproduced from* Phelan JP. Perinatal risk management: obstetric methods to prevent birth asphyxia. Clin Perinatol 2005;32:1–17; with permission.)

To illustrate the concept of notice or warning, an acute fetal distress pattern that arose without warning or in the absence of notice is illustrated in Fig. 4. Here, the FHR pattern is reactive with a normal baseline heart rate. Without warning, there is a sudden, rapid, and sustained deterioration of the FHR. In the absence of notice or warning, the risk management analysis or the litigation focus of the case will be on how well the obstetric team handled the resultant emergency.

In contrast, the fetal monitor strip for a patient who had a previous cesarean delivery is illustrated in Figs. 5 and 6. On admission to the hospital and before the start of the induction of labor, the patient has a reactive FHR pattern with a normal baseline rate. About 2 hours later, there is a sudden appearance of moderate or severe variable decelerations early in labor. The sudden appearance of moderate or severe variable decelerations in a patient

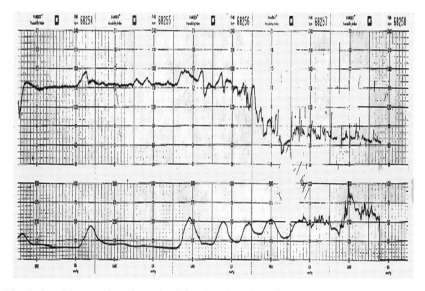

Fig. 4. A sudden, rapid, and sustained deterioration of the fetal heart rate in the absence of notice or warning. (*Reproduced from* Phelan JP. Perinatal risk management: obstetric methods to prevent birth asphyxia. Clin Perinatol 2005;32:1–17; with permission.)

A

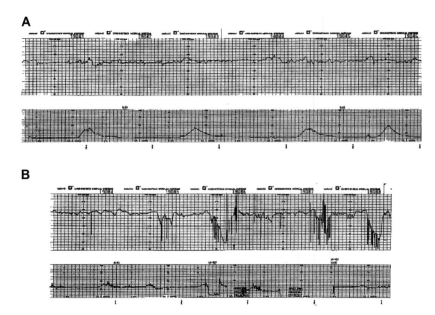

B

Fig. 5. (*A*) A patient is admitted at term with a history of a low transverse cesarean for induction of labor. (*B*) Approximately 2 hours later, the fetus develops a sudden increase in its baseline heart rate in association with moderate to severe variable decelerations early in labor. (*Reproduced from* Phelan JP. Perinatal risk management: obstetric methods to prevent birth asphyxia. Clin Perinatol 2005;32:1–17; with permission.)

who had a previous cesarean section at a time in labor when they are not anticipated can be a sign of uterine rupture [7]. The obstetric health care team is thus on notice of the potential for a uterine rupture or an abruption. With prompt recognition (see Fig. 6) in this case, the patient is seen in the operating room. Despite the uterine rupture, the patient had a favorable outcome.

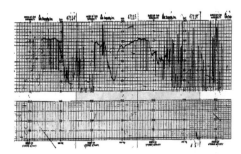

Fig. 6. The same case as in Fig. 5 is now in the operating room. The fetal heart rate has increased to about 180 bpm in association with severe variable decelerations. (*Reproduced from* Phelan JP. Perinatal risk management: obstetric methods to prevent birth asphyxia. Clin Perinatol 2005;32:1–17; with permission.)

Fetal brain injury

The global cerebral palsy (CP) rate (ie, the rate of all types of CP) is estimated to be approximately 1 to 2 cases per 1000 live births [8]. CP that is caused by hypoxic ischemic encephalopathy (HIE) in the singleton term infant is even rarer, with a reported prevalence of approximately 1 in 12,500 live births [9]. This rate has declined steadily over the last several decades [9,10]. Notwithstanding the decline and the rarity of this form of CP, there has been and continues to be a societal presumption that most, if not all, cases of HIE-induced CP occur during the 3 hours that are related to the events of labor and delivery. Unfortunately for the obstetric provider, society has tended to overlook the remaining 7000 hours of the pregnancy. As a result of this societal perspective, the obstetrician at times has been targeted unfairly as the person who is responsible for a given child's neurologic injuries. Nevertheless, numerous physicians and researchers have attempted to unravel the HIE-induced CP mystery [11,12]. To date, their efforts primarily have been limited to trying to classify fetal outcome based on birth-related endpoints [11] rather than looking at the continuum of fetal to neonatal life [12].

One aspect of the HIE-induced CP mystery is that its rarity has precluded in-depth studies into its pathogenesis. Until recently, little information has been available [12] to study these infants much beyond the moment of birth. As a result, many of the approaches to time or date of fetal brain injury have focused primarily on birth-related endpoints, such as the newborn's umbilical artery pH that is measured at the time of birth [11,13,14]. Rather, the entire pregnancy, labor, delivery, and well beyond birth require examination to understand fully the pathophysiologic mechanisms that are responsible for an infant's brain injuries and their long-term impact on the child. Critical to understanding the pathophysiology of HIE-induced CP is the ability to maintain an open mind when analyzing studies and not to prejudge them merely because they do not feed one's personal or scientific biases or are not considered mainstream at the time. Moreover, scientists know that under the HIE-induced CP umbrella, children manifest their asphyxial injury in various ways.

Scientists who have studied asphyxiated neonates realize that often times these babies were injured under vastly differing circumstances. For example, some may have been injured in the past and yet survived in utero to be live born; some may have been injured acutely intrapartum and likely would have died without intervention. Injured neonates may differ in their presentation because of differences in the timing, mechanism, or severity of the asphyxial episode. Our clinical understanding of this condition may not be improved by analyzing asphyxiated neonates as one group or under one umbrella. Phelan and Ahn [15] distinguished clinical patterns that were associated with term neonates who had permanent brain injury by using the admission intrapartum fetal heart rate (FHR) pattern. Although this classification cannot determine the exact moment when fetal brain injury occurred, this classification system does permit the identification of three groups of fetuses who were injured at different time intervals and in many cases in different ways. For example, Phelan and Ahn [15] showed that some infants were injured before presenting in labor, some were injured acutely during labor and delivered emergently, and some were injured during labor over some prolonged period of time before delivery. For that matter and with the exception of life expectancy, the following causation questions or issues are frequently asked in each and every case of a brain-damaged baby:

When did the asphyxial event begin?
What caused it to happen?
When did the brain injury occur?

Timing of fetal brain injury and fetal monitoring

Electronic fetal monitoring (EFM) has become an invaluable adjunct in the assessment of antepartum and intrapartum fetal well-being and serves a role in the timing of fetal brain injury. Since its inception, the goal of EFM has been to assess fetal health continually during labor and to permit the early detection of intrapartum fetal distress in sufficient time to theoretically prevent fetal brain injury. To achieve that goal, the presence of contraction-mediated FHR decelerations, such as repetitive or persistent late decelerations usually in conjunction with a loss of variability, has served as the basis for intervention. If traditional maneuvers of intrauterine resuscitation, such as maternal position change, oxygen administration, intravenous fluid administration, or discontinuance of oxytocin, failed to remedy the abnormal FHR pattern within a reasonable period of time, expedited delivery was indicated. Using this approach, the apparent benefit of continuous EFM has been limited to the reduction of intrapartum fetal deaths [16].

This trend is in keeping with the prescient observations of Perkins [17] almost 2 decades ago and was recently amplified in the Neonatal Encephalopathy Committee Opinion in 2003 (Box 1) [11]. For example, Perkins [17] opined that "the number of infants injured during labor is highly overestimated and the number injured before labor is highly underestimated." The prevailing belief then, and probably today [11], is that changes in the FHR preceded fetal neurologic impairment; however, as we have learned, not all fetuses undergo brain injury in such a manner [15,18]. As suggested by these clinical investigators, many fetuses present with preexisting neurologic impairment and their FHR patterns seem to be a manifestation of their underlying or preexisting brain damage. These researchers also suggested that fetal monitoring may be more helpful in identifying those fetuses who have already sustained central nervous system injury before admission to the hospital or to the obstetrician's office. To use EFM to prevent birth

---

Box 1. The Neonatal Encephalopathy Committee Opinion in 2003 criteria to define an acute intrapartum hypoxic event as sufficient to cause cerebral palsy

Essential criteria (must meet all four)

Evidence of a metabolic acidosis in fetal umbilical cord arterial blood obtained at delivery (pH <7 and base deficit ≥12 mmol/L).

Early onset of severe or moderate neonatal encephalopathy in infants born at 34 or more weeks of gestation.

Cerebral palsy of the spastic quadriplegic or dyskinetic type.

Exclusion of other identifiable causes, such as trauma, coagulation disorders, infectious conditions, or genetic disorders.

Nonessential criteria

Criteria that collectively suggest an intrapartum timing (within close proximity to labor and delivery (eg, 0–48 hours) but are nonspecific to asphyxial insults.

   A sentinel (signal) hypoxic event occurring immediately before or during labor.

   A sudden and sustained fetal bradycardia or the absence of FHR variability in the presence of persistent, late, or variable decelerations, usually after a hypoxic sentinel event when the pattern was previously normal.

   Apgar score of 0 to 3 beyond 5 minutes.

   Onset of multisystem involvement within 72 hours of birth.

   Early imaging study showing evidence of acute nonfocal cerebral abnormality

---

Data from Neonatal Encephalopathy Committee Opinion—2003: American College of Obstetricians and Gynecologists and The American Academy of Pediatrics. Washington, DC.

---

asphyxia, therefore, the clinician is left with the identification of the fetus who is at risk for asphyxia or is becoming asphyxiated. The continued reliance on contraction-mediated FHR decelerations in association with a loss of FHR variability as a clinical endpoint, although considered by some to be mainstream, does not take into account the concepts of foreseeability of harm, notice, the window to fetal brain injury, and potentially preventable fetal brain injury. To determine whether fetal brain injury is potentially preventable requires a separate analysis beyond mere identification and an earlier delivery and must also satisfy a reasonableness test.

Determining the timing of fetal brain injury is a highly complex issue. Before an obstetric expert can consider whether the fetal brain injury was potentially preventable, one must be able to determine whether the fetus was already injured on admission to the hospital or to the obstetrician's office. After that initial assessment, one can then determine whether the fetus is at risk for asphyxia or is becoming asphyxiated. Then the analysis necessarily switches to determine whether the fetal brain injury was or is potentially preventable.

The first step in any causation analysis is to determine whether the fetus is or is not, in all medical probability or certainty, neurologically normal on admission to the hospital or the physician's office. The fetal or labor admission test can serve as the basis for that initial assessment [19]. Although the clinical goals of the labor admission test are to identify those fetuses who are at risk for intrapartum fetal distress and to reassign those patients who are alleged to be at high or low risk before labor to a different risk category soon after admission to labor and delivery, the use of the initial admission test or fetal monitoring period is also helpful in a causation analysis for purposes of timing fetal brain injury. If, for example, the patient's FHR pattern on admission to the hospital is considered to be reactive, labor and delivery personnel know that the fetus is probably, but not absolutely, normal [20]. In this case one would not be able to apply the legal standard of "beyond a reasonable doubt" to a reactive admission FHR pattern because a fetus who had anencephaly, hydrocephaly, or preexisting basal ganglia injury could have a reactive FHR pattern on admission to the hospital [20]. Labor and delivery personnel also recognize that the presence of a reactive fetal admission test is a sign of a healthy fetus and symbolizes fetal well-being, normal fetal acid–base status, normoxia and absence of asphyxia, and a low probability of intrapartum fetal distress [12,19]. When timing fetal brain injury, the application of the legal standard of "in all medical probability or certainty" to a reactive admission FHR pattern means that the fetus is, in all medical probability or certainty, neurologically normal.

In contrast, a nonreactive fetal admission test or the absence of FHR accelerations is associated with a greater probability of an adverse outcome. If, for example, the fetus on admission to the hospital has persistent fetal nonreactivity, or is unable to generate a spontaneous or evoked FHR acceleration for more than 120 minutes from the time of admission to the hospital, increased rates of perinatal mortality and permanent neurologic impairment are observed [2,3,19]. In essence, and unlike the fetus who has a reactive FHR pattern on admission, the fetus who has a persistent nonreactive FHR pattern is in all medical probability or certainty neurologically impaired. The obstetric provider could not, in most if not all instances, have prevented the brain injury after admission to the hospital. The primary reason is that one cannot prevent that which has already happened.

To illustrate this concept, Figs. 7 and 8 demonstrate the same fetus 3 days apart. In Fig. 7 (Time A), the fetus has a reactive FHR monitor strip and normal fetal movement. At Time A, a reasonable obstetric expert could conclude that the fetus was, to a degree of medical probability or certainty,

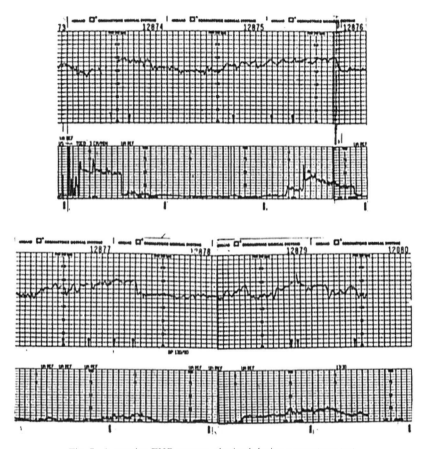

Fig. 7. A reactive FHR pattern obtained during a nonstress test.

neurologically normal. When the mother returns 3 days later, (Time B; see Fig. 8), the fetus has a persistent nonreactive FHR pattern and is no longer able to accelerate its heart rate. In addition, the fetus is noted to have decreased or absent fetal movement for the 24 hours before admission to the hospital at Time B. At the end of the fetal monitor strip at Time B, the fetus was delivered. At some time after delivery, the fetus was noted to have spastic quadriplegia.

Clearly, the fetus at Time A (see Fig. 7) is distinguishable from the fetus we see at Time B (see Fig. 8). Based on these observed changes, several questions come to mind. The obvious first question is, what happened during those 3 days? How and why did this fetal heart rate change so dramatically in just 3 days? How did this child become brain damaged? When the two figures are compared two important fetal monitoring issues are demonstrated in Fig. 8: (1) there was no evidence of uterine activity, (2) there were no late decelerations. In fact, the only FHR decelerations were two

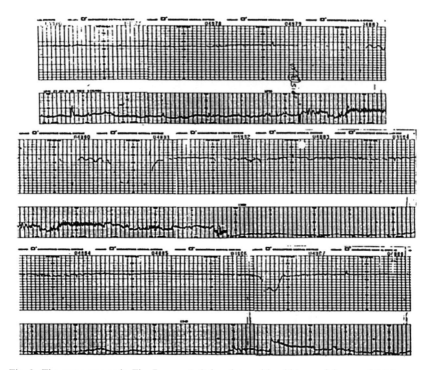

Fig. 8. The same case as in Fig. 7 presents 3 days later with a history of decreased fetal movement for 24 hours. A persistent nonreactive FHR pattern with two variable FHR decelerations is observed on the fetal monitor strip.

Krebs and colleagues [21] atypical variable decelerations ("W" pattern) on the fetal monitor strip. Based on those two observations, two important questions should be asked. First, if contractions are the mediator of fetal harm, how was this child injured during the period from Time A to Time B without uterine contractions? Second, if repetitive or persistent late or variable decelerations represent the final endpoint as it relates to causing fetal brain injury, where are the persistent late or variable decelerations?

With that as a backdrop, an analysis of the hypothetical case in Figs. 7 and 8 would be helpful to further our understanding of the role of causation in a brain-injured baby case. In this case, we are limited to the two FHR patterns and the maternal history of decreased or absent fetal movement for the 24 hours before the maternal admission at Time B. At Time A, the fetus was, in all medical probability or certainty, neurologically normal. Between Time A and Time B, there was the development of decreased or absent fetal movement. At the moment of maternal admission to the hospital and placement of the fetal monitor, a persistent nonreactive FHR pattern without any FHR accelerations was recorded. This finding, in addition to the other findings, would be consistent with preexisting fetal brain injury. Because the fetus on admission to the hospital at Time B had preexisting neurologic impairment, the causation nexus (see Fig. 1) for the intrapartum obstetric care would be broken and the bridge between any alleged breach in the standard of obstetric care and the fetal brain damage would obviously collapse. This finding also means that the fetus could not have been made whole with earlier intervention at Time B. If, for example, a cesarean section was done at the moment the mother presented to the hospital, the fetus would not, in all medical probability or certainty, have been neurologically normal.

The remaining medical–legal questions relate to whether there is evidence of an ongoing asphyxia or a secondary fetal brain injury at Time B. For this case, the answer to those questions is probably not. Before we address those questions further, we next explore the current approaches to time fetal brain injury.

Current approaches to time fetal brain injury

For centuries, scientists have attempted to establish various ways to time fetal brain injury. At first, attention was focused on the several hours during which a patient was in labor. It was for this reason that electronic fetal monitoring was invented. The operant presumption has been that the intrapartum FHR pattern would theoretically alert the obstetrician in sufficient time to prevent fetal brain injury caused by HIE. One must ask what went wrong. Was there a failure of fetal monitoring or was it something else? First, our fetal monitoring forefathers underestimated the number of infants who were injured before labor and overestimated the number who were injured during labor [12]. At best, the fetal monitor permitted us to prevent intrapartum deaths [16]. As a result, some neonates were able to survive, albeit in an impaired state. One must consider whether the birth of such children was a failure of fetal monitoring or a failure to recognize a fetus who had preexisting neurologic impairment [12]. Gaziano and Freeman [22] wrote in 1977 that "in the adult, fixed heart rate patterns are associated with severe central nervous system injury. In the fetus …this pattern may be the end result of [a] severe CNS hypoxic insult." The pattern described by Gaziano and Freeman [22] is similar to the FHR pattern observed in Fig. 8. One cannot prevent that which has already been damaged. It also follows that the obstetrician should not be faulted in that circumstance for any resultant neurologic impairment. This reasoning begs the question of whether the failures of fetal monitoring are related to the current approaches to the interpretation of fetal monitoring [23] or to the presumption that the use of the fetal monitor should result in the prevention of CP through earlier detection and timely intervention. Before one can prevent a neurologic insult, one must be able to identify which fetus is at risk for that brain damage and then make a determination of whether that insult is potentially preventable.

Two approaches [11,12] have emerged to assist us with the timing of fetal brain injury. One approach was developed by the Neonatal Encephalopathy

Committee (NEC) of the American College of Obstetricians and Gynecologists (ACOG) and the American Academy of Pediatrics (Table 1) [11] and
the other [12] by the Childbirth Injury Prevention Foundation (Childbirth)
(Box 2). Neither approach is perfect, but both approaches represent valiant attempts to address the highly complex issue of timing fetal brain damage.

The Neonatal Encephalopathy Committee Opinion of 2003 [11] used
ACOG 163 [13] and the International Consensus Criteria [14] to form the
foundation for this new approach. A clear benefit of the NEC approach
[11] was the injection of a fifth clause that excluded many fetal brain injuries
unrelated to HIE from the analysis (see Table 1). As with the early approaches, the emphasis was on the events that surrounded birth, including
metabolic acidemia on an umbilical artery cord gas and the presence of neonatal encephalopathy. The ongoing dilemma with this approach is the requirement of metabolic acidemia to determine whether an insult occurred
intrapartum. The likelihood of permanent neurologic impairment in neonates who have severe acidosis at birth is uncommon and is estimated to
be approximately 8% to 9% [24]. Volpe's [25] textbook, *Neurology of the
Newborn*, commented on an article regarding the relationship between metabolic acidosis and long-term neurologic impairment and noted that "approximately 85% of the asphyxiated neonates either were normal or
exhibited minor deficits at 1 year of age" [26].

The Childbirth approach is a flexible method to time fetal brain injury.
This overall approach captures the key elements of fetal life and incorporates the essential ingredients of the neonatal period. The mainstay of the
Childbirth method is the use of the intrapartum FHR pattern. The underlying rationale for using the intrapartum FHR pattern is that fetuses who become or have been brain damaged manifest their injuries in consistent ways
on the fetal monitor strip. Based on the work of Phelan and Ahn [15,18],
these distinct intrapartum FHR patterns are linked to findings in the neonatal period and the location of the fetal brain injury [27,28]. As demonstrated
in Box 2, the Childbirth approach uses fetal and neonatal findings to time
fetal brain injury. The fetal findings include the admission FHR pattern,

Table 1
The Childbirth Injury Prevention Foundation's flexible method to time fetal brain injury is
demonstrated [12]

FHR pattern	B	NRBC count
Fetal movement	I	NRBC clearance time
	R	Platelet count
	T	Seizure onset
	H	Organ dysfunction
		Brain injury location
Fetal period		Neonatal period

Abbreviations: FHR, fetal heart rate; NRBC, nucleated red blood cell.
Data from Phelan JP, Kim JO. Fetal heart rate observations in the brain-damaged infant.
Semin Perinatol 2000;24:221–9.

Box 2. The window to fetal brain injury may be affected by one or more of these factors

Previous FHR pattern
Fetal growth
Degree of intrafetal shunting
Duration of the deceleration
Intactness of the placenta

Data from Phelan JP. Perinatal risk management: obstetric methods to prevent birth asphyxia. Clin Perinatol 2005;32:1–17.

---

the characteristics of fetal movement on admission, and the subsequent changes in the intrapartum FHR pattern, if any, during labor and delivery. The neonatal findings include but are not limited to hematologic markers, such as nucleated red blood cells (NRBC), the NRBC clearance times, platelet counts, liver enzymes, changes in the serum sodium [29,30], the onset of neonatal seizures, neuroimaging for the location of the brain damage, and the long-term follow-up of the child. All of these neonatal findings have been linked scientifically to the intrapartum FHR pattern [3,12].

The Childbirth approach is analogous to viewing an impressionist painting. You must look at the entire painting to understand its overall significance and not limit your visual perspective to a postage stamp area of the painting. For example, you cannot use NRBC values alone to time fetal brain injury. In timing fetal brain injury, the Childbirth approach is also not limited to the findings that surround the moment of birth, such as umbilical artery cord gases and Apgar scores, but focuses on the continuum of life and the transition from fetal to neonatal life and beyond [3,12]. Simply stated, the Childbirth approach requires visualization of the entire painting to understand the timing of a given child's fetal brain injury.

When the two approaches to time fetal brain injury are compared, the methods have many similarities. For example, each approach focuses on hypoxic ischemic encephalopathy as the basis for the CP, such as the type of cerebral palsy (spastic quadriplegia or athetoid or dyskinetic cerebral palsy [NEC]) or the location of the brain injury (Childbirth). This distinction is important because certain FHR patterns, as shown by other researchers [28] and the Childbirth research group [2,3,12,27], give rise to brain injury in specific areas of the fetal brain. For example, a fetus who has a sudden, rapid, and sustained deterioration of the FHR that is unresponsive to remedial measures or terbutaline and lasts for a prolonged period of time typically sustains in an injury to the basal ganglia or the deep gray matter that gives rise to athetoid or dyskinetic cerebral palsy [2,3,12,27,28]. In this case the brain injury is the result of a sudden reduction of fetal cardiac output and blood pressure or "cerebral hypotension due to an ineffective or nonfunctional cardiac pump" usually

following a sentinel hypoxic event, such as a uterine rupture or a cord prolapse. That is not to say that the fetus cannot have injury to both the deep
gray matter and the cerebral hemispheres with this FHR pattern. Whether
both areas of the fetal brain are affected often depends on the five factors illustrated in Box 2. In contrast, the persistent nonreactive FHR pattern character-
istically results in damage to both cerebral hemispheres and give rise to spastic
quadriplegia [2,3,12,27]. Here the mechanism for injury is not an ineffective
pump, because these fetuses usually demonstrate normal baseline heart rates
but without FHR accelerations. The brain damage in this situation relates
more to cerebral ischemia.

One of the key differences between these two approaches is that the
Childbirth approach is broader and attempts to focus on the timing of fetal
brain injury before and after hospital admission based on the characteristics
of the admission and subsequent intrapartum FHR patterns. The NEC approach clearly focuses on the intrapartum period, and would be comparable
to the Childbirth study population with a reactive FHR pattern at the time
of hospital admission followed by a sudden, rapid, and sustained deterioration of the fetal heart rate usually attributable to a sentinel hypoxic event. In
keeping with that approach, the NEC emphasizes and the Childbirth approach de-emphasizes the events surrounding birth as a means to time fetal
brain injury, such as umbilical arterial cord blood gases, Apgar scores, and
Sarnat criteria for neonatal encephalopathy. Both, however, arrive at the
same conclusion as to the timing of the fetal brain injury during the intrapartum period [31]. The Childbirth approach, when applied to the fetus
with a reactive FHR pattern at the time of hospital admission followed
by a sudden, rapid, and sustained deterioration of the FHR unresponsive
to remedial measures usually attributable to a sentinel hypoxic event, also
presumes metabolic acidemia (umbilical artery cord blood gas pH <7.00
and a base deficit >12 mmol/L), moderate or severe neonatal encephalopathy, and spastic quadriplegia or dyskinetic cerebral palsy [31]. The Childbirth approach arrives at the same conclusion as to the timing of the
brain injury by using other neonatal factors, such as the NRBC counts
and clearance times, the initial platelet count, the onset of neonatal seizures,
the degree of organ dysfunction, and the location of the brain damage. Once
again, the key distinction is that the Childbirth approach is an effort to incorporate all the different ways a fetus can become brain damaged into one
overall approach to time fetal brain injury. Regardless of the approach used
to time fetal brain injury, it is amazingly clear that the efforts of both groups
are designed to provide families of children who have CP with a greater
understanding of what happened to their child.

Fetal brain injury cases—a causation analysis

This section of the article reviews a causation analysis of several hypothetical cases. To begin this analysis, we use the case demonstrated in

Figs. 7 and 8. The fetus had a reactive strip 3 days before maternal admission to the hospital. Then the mother experienced decreased or absent fetal movement 24 hours before admission. On placement of the fetal monitor, a persistent nonreactive FHR pattern was observed with a baseline rate at or around 160 beats per minute (bpm). Soon after admission, the fetus was delivered and no sentinel hypoxic event was identified. Umbilical artery cord blood gases were normal and without evidence of metabolic acidemia. After birth, the neonate developed seizures (moderate encephalopathy). Later the neonate was diagnosed with spastic quadriplegic cerebral palsy and cortical blindness because of HIE and without any identifiable genetic abnormality.

The application of either approach to this case would give the same result, that this neonate's brain injury did not happen intrapartum but was an injury that, in all medical probability or certainty, preceded maternal admission to the hospital. For example, the application of the NEC criteria to this case would demonstrate that the essential element of metabolic acidemia based on an abnormal umbilical artery cord gas was not present. If an umbilical artery cord blood gas was not obtained at birth, however, the neonate would, in all medical probability or certainty, have a normal umbilical artery cord gas because the fetus at the time of birth did not have a slow heart rate [32]. On quick analysis, the NEC nonessential criteria for heart rate and a sentinel hypoxic event would also not be satisfied. The timing of the fetal brain injury would thus fall outside the intrapartum period.

Based on the persistent nonreactive FHR pattern (see Fig. 8) and the maternal history of decreased or absent fetal movement 24 hours before hospital admission, the application of the Childbirth criteria would also suggest a preadmission and not an intrapartum injury. Here is where the two approaches diverge. As illustrated in Table 2, the Childbirth approach incorporates several neonatal parameters to augment or explain the timing of fetal brain injury. With the application of the Childbirth criteria (see Table 1) and the factors identified in Table 2, the fetus would be classified as having sustained its brain injury before maternal admission to the hospital.

A few physicians might ask if there is evidence for ongoing asphyxia in Fig. 8. If there was ongoing injury, what would you expect to see on the fetal

Table 2
Hypothetical neonatal findings

Neonatal study	Result
NRBC count	52 %
NRBC clearance time	145 hours
Initial platelet count	95,000/μL
Seizure onset	18 hours after birth
Organ dysfunction	Liver, kidneys, bone marrow, lungs, heart
Brain injury location	Bilateral cerebral hemispheres

Abbreviation: NRBC, nucleated red blood cells (number/100 white blood cells).

monitor strip? Fetuses who are undergoing progressive asphyxia, according to Hon [2,12,15], manifest a progressive and continuous increase in the baseline heart rate in association with repetitive FHR decelerations and usually a loss of variability. In this case the fetal monitor strip demonstrates a baseline rate at or around 160 bpm and probably diminished FHR variability, but we do not see a progressive and continuous increase in the baseline rate, and, of note clinically, there were no repetitive or persistent FHR decelerations. The baseline FHR remained fixed and there were solely two variable decelerations. In the absence of a sudden, rapid, and sustained deterioration of the FHR, or the "Hon changes," there was, in all medical probability or certainty, no secondary fetal brain injury or ongoing fetal asphyxia in this case.

Fig. 9 illustrates a case similar to the one in Fig. 8, but with a sustained deterioration of the FHR at the end of the fetal monitor strip that lasted until delivery. Once again we have a persistent nonreactive FHR pattern and decreased or absent fetal movement for 18 hours this time rather than 24 hours. In contrast with the case in Fig. 8, there is a sustained deterioration of the FHR at the end of the fetal monitor strip that continues through to the delivery of the fetus. Unlike the fetus in Fig. 8, this fetus had, in all medical probability or certainty, a metabolic acidemia with an umbilical artery cord blood pH <7.00 and a base deficit >12 mmol/L. During the neonatal

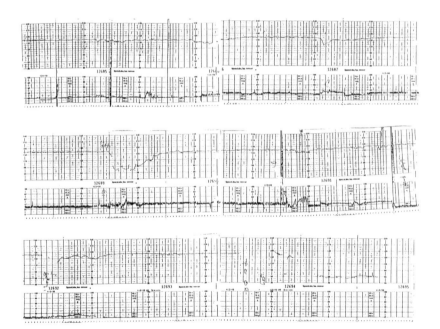

Fig. 9. A case is presented with a history of decreased fetal movement for 18 hours. On placement of the fetal monitor, a persistent nonreactive FHR pattern is observed for a period of time and is followed by sudden, rapid, and sustained deterioration of the FHR that lasts until delivery.

period the fetus had moderate encephalopathy and on long-term follow-up was diagnosed with spastic quadriplegia and cortical blindness. No genetic or inherited disorders were identified. Does the presence of metabolic acidemia now mean that the fetus in Fig. 9 sustained its brain damage intrapartum as opposed to preadmission? With the addition of metabolic acidemia, the NEC essential criteria are apparently satisfied. As a result, the NEC essential and nonessential criteria would seem to place the timing of the injury during the intrapartum period.

A respectable number of clinicians might ask if the nonessential requirement that the sustained deterioration of the FHR in a fetus with a previously normal pattern was satisfied. The Childbirth approach requires a reactive FHR pattern on admission for the classification of normal. In Fig. 9, the previous or admission FHR pattern would not be considered previously normal because of the persistently nonreactive FHR pattern. Conversely, a few physicians might argue that because of the vagueness or the overbroad nature of the term "previously normal," the admission FHR pattern was in fact normal because there was a normal baseline rate. As such, the NEC approach [11] might theoretically apply, and, once again, place the timing of the fetal brain injury during the intrapartum period.

In contrast, the Childbirth approach would clearly time the brain damage before maternal admission to the hospital because of the persistent nonreactive FHR pattern and the presence of decreased or absent fetal movement. Additionally, if we assume that the fetus had the same neonatal findings as illustrated in Table 2, in which the fetus had an elevated NRBC count and a prolonged NRBC clearance time, a low initial platelet count, a similar degree of organ dysfunction, seizure onset, and brain injury location, the timing of the fetal brain injury would fall outside the window of care.

The sole remaining question for the fetus in Fig. 9 is whether the fetus sustained a secondary injury as a consequence of the sustained deterioration of the FHR before delivery or if the fetal brain damage was limited to a single injury. Obviously, whether the fetus did sustain secondary brain damage would depend to a certain extent on the five factors previously identified in Box 2 and whether the fetus, as a result of the slow heart rate before delivery, sustained a deep gray-matter injury that was confirmed with neuroimaging. If there was a basal ganglia injury, the question that would still need to be asked is if the basal ganglia injury represents a secondary injury. The ongoing conflict here is whether the injury arose before or after maternal admission to the hospital. If all the brain damage arose intrapartum, the brain-injured child can theoretically be made whole. If the brain injury is shown by a preponderance of the evidence to have occurred preadmission, the brain-damaged child cannot be made whole.

We are thus back to the question of whether there was a secondary injury. In the absence of well-defined and confirmed deep gray-matter injury, a reasonable scientific conclusion would be that there was a single injury and that injury predated maternal admission to the hospital. If neuroimaging confirmed a basal ganglia injury, the factors in Box 2 and specifically the duration of the sustained deterioration of the fetal heart rate would have to be taken into consideration. Assuming one can then link the basal ganglia injury to the intrapartum period, the resultant brain injury would then be considered secondary and not primary.

But that is not the end of the analysis. One must still make a separate determination of whether the secondary basal ganglia injury was in fact potentially preventable. A two-prong analysis of the obstetric care would be obstetrically necessary. The first question would be if there was sufficient notice to the physician and nursing personnel that the FHR was, to a degree of medical probability or certainty, going to crash. The second analytical step would be to determine how well they handled the obstetric emergency once the FHR did crash. To conduct the analysis, we assume the basal ganglia injury was determined to be a secondary injury that occurred intrapartum and did not arise before maternal admission to the hospital. To answer the question of notice, one must ask whether a persistent nonreactive FHR pattern by itself constituted sufficient notice that the crash was going to occur. If the persistent nonreactive FHR pattern does not constitute sufficient notice to the providers of the potential for a crash in the FHR, the focus shifts to the handling of the emergency after the FHR crashed to show, to a degree of medical probability, that the basal ganglia injury was potentially preventable with an earlier delivery.

Even if we assume that the basal ganglia injury to this fetus was potentially preventable, the next analytic step would be to apportion the primary and secondary brain injuries. For illustrative purposes solely, the primary injury could be apportioned as being responsible for 75% of the child's current condition and the basal ganglia or secondary injury would be apportioned to the remaining 25%. In this theoretical situation this means that the injured child could not be returned to whole and recovery would be limited to 25%. In other words, the 25% would represent the portion of the child's brain damage related to the negligent care during labor and delivery.

Causation also relates to not only the timing and prevention of fetal brain injury but also to the potential prevention of fetal death. Figs. 10 and 11 illustrate the unique stair-steps to heaven or death intrapartum FHR pattern (Table 3). This rare FHR pattern was first described by Hon [33] as a decreasing baseline rate and later by Krebs and colleagues [34] as a progressive bradycardia. The characteristics of the stair-steps to heaven intrapartum FHR pattern are as follows:

A persistent nonreactive FHR pattern without FHR accelerations.
From the time of maternal admission to the hospital there is a gradual reduction or decline in the baseline FHR over time usually in 5 to 10 bpm increments. Once the FHR reaches 90 to 100 bpm, the FHR is usually lost.
FHR decelerations are usually absent.

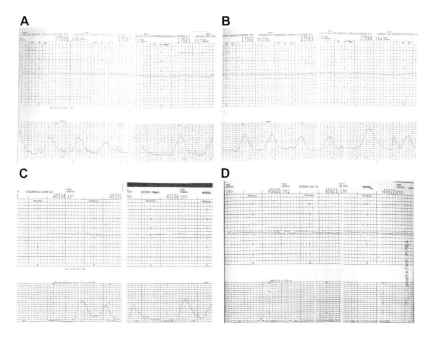

Fig. 10. (A) This case presents in labor with a persistent nonreactive FHR pattern and a baseline FHR of 135 bpm. (B) The FHR pattern remains persistently nonreactive with a baseline FHR of 135 bpm. (C) The FHR pattern remains persistently nonreactive and the baseline FHR is now 130 bpm. (D) The FHR pattern remains persistently nonreactive and the baseline FHR is now 125 bpm.

As demonstrated in Figs. 10 and 11, the FHR starts at 135 bpm on admission. Over the period of monitoring, the baseline heart rate gradually declines from the initial rate of 135 bpm (see Fig. 10A) in 5 to 10 bpm increments to 100 bpm. Then the FHR is lost (see Fig. 11D). Note that there were no FHR decelerations during the entire period of fetal monitoring. This FHR pattern is associated with a high perinatal mortality rate and the survivors are typically severely impaired neurologically (see Table 2). The high cesarean delivery rate in this population of almost 87% did not prevent the death or permanent disability of these fetuses.

The stair-steps to heaven or death intrapartum FHR pattern is rare. If, for example, the incidence of HIE-induced cerebral palsy ranges from 1/4000 births [35] to 1/12,500 births [9], the incidence of this FHR pattern ranges from 1/61,000 births to 1/190,000 births. If your hospital does 3000 deliveries a year, it is estimated that you will see this FHR pattern on labor and delivery once every 20.3 to 63.3 years.

The causation argument in these cases focuses on whether an earlier cesarean delivery would, in all medical probability or certainty, have resulted in a neurologically normal child. Once again, the causation analysis begins with the admission FHR pattern. In this case the FHR pattern was

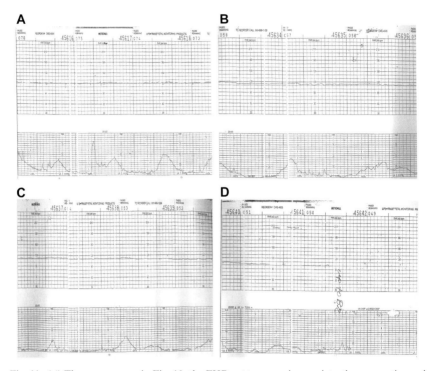

Fig. 11. (A) The same case as in Fig. 10; the FHR pattern remains persistently nonreactive and the baseline FHR is now 120 bpm. (B) The FHR pattern remains persistently nonreactive and the baseline FHR is now 115 bpm. (C) The FHR pattern remains persistently nonreactive and the baseline FHR is now 110 bpm. (D) The FHR pattern remains persistently nonreactive and the baseline FHR is now 100 bpm. Then the FHR is lost.

persistently nonreactive without evidence of FHR accelerations or decelerations. As we learned earlier, the fetus was, in all medical probability or certainty, permanently neurologically impaired from the moment of maternal admission to the hospital. A cesarean delivery performed at the moment of maternal admission to the hospital would not have resulted in a child who would, in all medical probability or certainty, have been born neurologically normal.

The major question raised by this intrapartum FHR pattern is not whether earlier delivery would have resulted in a neurologically normal child, but whether the fetus will, in all medical probability or certainty, be born alive and survive, albeit in an impaired state. The dilemma is that when we monitor the fetus in Figs. 10 and 11, the fetus, by virtue of the intrapartum FHR pattern, is telling us that he or she is in the process of dying. Although cesarean section did seem to prevent death in some fetuses, the 26 (68%) survivors with this FHR pattern did have significant permanent neurologic impairment. This finding would seem to support the observations of Yeh and associates [16] that the fetal monitor does

Table 3
Perinatal outcome for 38 fetuses who had stair-steps to heaven intrapartum FHR pattern

Factor	Number (%)
DFM documented	9 (24)
Sentinel hypoxic event	6 (16)
Meconium	27 (71)
Cesarean section	33 (87)
Perinatal deaths	12 (32)

Abbreviation: DFM, decreased fetal movement.

afford us the ability to prevent intrapartum death through intervention but does not afford us the opportunity to prevent preexisting neurologic impairment.

At the beginning of this article, the discussion centered on the concept of notice and a description of what constitutes intrapartum fetal distress with (see Figs. 5 and 6) and without notice or warning (see Fig. 4). Continuing with Justice Cardozo's concept of foreseeability of harm, Figs. 12 and 13A and B illustrate a gravida who presented for induction of labor because

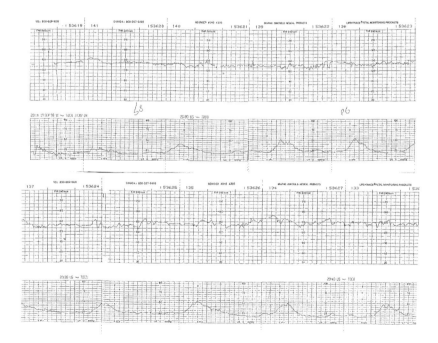

Fig. 12. This case represents an admission for induction of labor because of suspected oligohydramnios with an amniotic fluid index of 1.0 cm. At the time of maternal admission the FHR pattern is reactive.

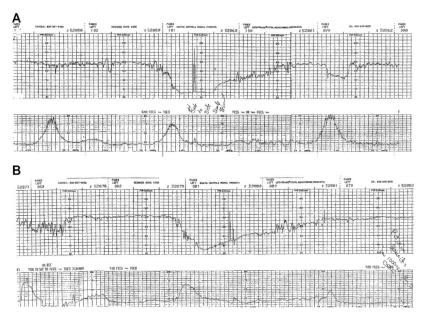

Fig. 13. (*A*) The same case as in Fig. 12; the FHR pattern continues to be reactive but three FHR decelerations are observed. One FHR deceleration lasts about 5 to 6 minutes. (*B*) At a later time, two additional FHR decelerations are observed with one lasting 5 to 6 minutes.

of suspected oligohydramnios (amniotic fluid index equal to 1.0 cm). On maternal admission to the hospital, the fetus had a reactive FHR pattern and exhibited normal fetal movement. Using a causation analysis, the fetus was, in all medical probability or certainty, neurologically normal on maternal admission. As such, if the fetus does become brain damaged intrapartum the fetus has to demonstrate a Hon pattern of intrapartum ischemia or a sudden, rapid, and sustained deterioration of the fetal heart rate unresponsive to remedial measures or terbutaline [2,12,15,20].

At the time of maternal admission we also know that there was oligohydramnios and probably meconium-stained amniotic fluid [19,36]. Based on the finding of probable oligohydramnios, the fetus is undergoing intrafetal shunting and is at risk for umbilical cord compression. Intrafetal shunting means that the fetus is preferentially shunting blood away from organs, such as the kidneys and liver, to the fetal brain. In this case, the presence of oligohydramnios is an indicator of fetal blood flow being diverted away from the fetal kidneys. As a consequence of the oligohydramnios, therefore, it would be reasonably foreseeable that the fetus could theoretically crash during a trial of labor and become brain damaged. Using the five factors illustrated in Box 2, the fetus in Figs. 12 and 13 would, in the event of a crash in the FHR, be more like to sustain fetal brain injury earlier than the fetus who did not have intrafetal shunting and who had a normal amniotic fluid volume. Because of that foreseeable risk, the clinician could either heighten the level of intrapartum scrutiny in the event of the fetal potential to crash during the index labor or perform a cesarean to avoid the potential for the crash altogether.

When the fetus manifests an FHR deceleration for around 6 minutes (Fig. 13A) would that FHR deceleration constitute notice to the obstetric provider that the fetus has, in all medical probability or certainty, the potential to crash at some later time during the labor? After this 6-minute FHR deceleration, the clinical question would be if the labor should continue. When exercising medical judgment in that situation, it is important to remind ourselves that vaginal birth is not always the goal. The goal of any pregnancy is a healthy mother and baby. If the labor continues and the fetus does have a sudden, rapid, and sustained deterioration of the fetal heart rate, and as a result of that prolonged FHR deceleration the fetus sustains permanent brain damaged to the deep gray matter, could it be said that the crash and subsequent permanent neurologic impairment were reasonably foreseeable, and thus potentially preventable? It may be that in this clinical circumstance, the exercise of good medical judgment would permit continued labor so long as a physician capable of performing a cesarean section is immediately available. Assuming the labor does continue and the fetus sustains a second prolonged FHR deceleration (see Fig. 13B), would that be a sufficient indicator to terminate the labor because of the fetal potential to crash? If the labor continues and the fetus does have a sudden, rapid, and sustained deterioration of the FHR that lasts until delivery and does sustain permanent brain damage, it is easy to understand how Justice Cardozo's concept of foreseeability of harm and notice could apply in a brain-damaged baby case.

Although a few physicians may attempt to argue that the timing of the fetal brain injury predated maternal admission to the hospital because of the presence of intrafetal shunting (oligohydramnios and probable meconium), the NEC and Childbirth approaches to time fetal brain damage would, in all medical probability or certainty, categorize the brain damage as occurring intrapartum. The key to understanding this case is not how the NEC and Childbirth approaches would link the fetal brain damage to the intrapartum period; the key is to understand the foreseeable consequences of a gravida with oligohydramnios who has this intrapartum FHR pattern. Clearly, intervention in the form of a cesarean before the crash would have resulted, in all medical probability or certainty, in a neurologically normal child. The concept of foreseeability of harm serves to alert us, in selected cases, of the potential of the downstream consequence of a fetal bradycardia (see Figs. 3 and 13) and an opportunity to potentially prevent fetal brain injury.

Uterine rupture as a cause of fetal brain injury

Causation encompasses not only the timing of fetal brain injury but also the concept of what, if anything, is responsible for a uterine rupture. For example, Figs. 5 and 6 illustrate a prior cesarean patient who sustained a uterine rupture during an induction of labor. If she has a brain-damaged infant, the medical–legal focus is on not only the timely diagnosis of uterine rupture but also the cause of the uterine rupture. If there was an identifiable cause for a uterine rupture, the clinician should have avoided it, whatever it was, and the uterine rupture should never have happened. The medical–legal focus as to the cause of the uterine rupture is usually on whether the uses of oxytocin or cervical ripening agents or uterine activity patterns caused the uterine rupture and whether an intrauterine pressure catheter (IUPC) would have assisted in the earlier identification of a pending uterine rupture. Clearly, induction of labor with or without cervical ripening agents, and not augmentation of labor in a VBAC patient, is associated with a greater risk for uterine rupture [37]. The clinical dilemma is not whether there is a higher risk for uterine rupture in the prior cesarean patient. Gravidas with a prior cesarean section are significantly more likely to have a uterine rupture than gravidas without a history of a prior cesarean section [38]. The clinical difficulty is who, among the induction group or any VBAC, will actually sustain a ruptured uterus. Before the start of the VBAC clinicians do not have sufficient scientific evidence to say who will or will not rupture their uterus during a planned VBAC. This observation is true regardless of whether the VBAC patient does or does not receive oxytocin or any other agent [37,38]. Clinicians thus are left with attempting to identify, if possible, those VBAC patients who are experiencing a uterine rupture or to perform cesarean sections on all of them without a trial of labor.

What scientific evidence is there that the mere use of oxytocin or similar agents cause uterine rupture? If oxytocin is a proximate cause of uterine rupture, why does a patient who does not receive oxytocin or cervical ripening agents still rupture her uterus? In those patients who choose to undergo a VBAC, does the use of an intrauterine pressure catheter assist the clinician in readily diagnosing a uterine rupture? During that labor are there specific uterine activity patterns, such as uterine hyperstimulation, or tetanic episodes that cause or are associated with a uterine rupture? Based on available scientific evidence, an intrauterine pressure catheter does not assist in the diagnosis or identification of a uterine rupture [7]. The reason is that the uterus continues to contract after the uterus ruptures and there is not a loss of uterine tone or uterine activity [7]. Moreover, Phelan and associates [39] have shown in a case-controlled study that uterine hyperstimulation and tetanic episodes with or without the use of oxytocin were not markers for a pending uterine rupture, nor were these uterine activity patterns associated with an increased risk for uterine rupture. Moreover, these investigators [39] were also able to show that the uterine rupture group had significantly fewer contraction than did the two groups who did not have a uterine rupture.

The real problem is, however, which VBAC patient with or without an induction is actually going to rupture her uterus. Assuming an induction does go forward, as it did in Fig. 5, how are you going to identify the

VBAC patient who is rupturing her uterus? According to Rodriguez and associates [7], the single most reliable way for obstetric providers to identify that a VBAC patient is experiencing a uterine rupture is the sudden appearance of moderate or severe variable decelerations, as demonstrated in Figs. 5 and 6, at a time in labor when they are not expected. When the VBAC patient is at the end of the first stage or in the second stage of labor, the diagnosis of uterine rupture is clearly more difficult, if not impossible, because of the well-known changes in the FHR that accompany this period of labor.

As to the cause of uterine rupture, nobody knows for sure. It is easier to say what does not cause a uterine rupture than what actually causes it. Scientifically, the issue seems to relate to the placenta and its implantation site [40], the unfavorable cervix [37], or to a certain extent the embryologic development of the uterus itself. Continued exploration into these areas should ultimately bear fruit and also provide insights into this complicated and often tragic obstetric emergency.

The depressed neonate

Whenever a depressed neonate is delivered the obstetric concerns frequently turn to the question of why and how this happened. In most cases the obstetric providers will not be able to explain what happened for a considerable period of time after the child's birth because scientific data need to be gathered. This is especially true in the situation of a fetal death; the results of an autopsy may not be available for several weeks. We therefore need to become crime scene investigators (CSIs) when the depressed neonate is born and with the other members of the obstetric team gather and document the following scientific data in the medical records:

Maternal Kleihauer-Betke (KB) test
Admission fetal movement characteristics
Umbilical cord blood data
Placental pathology
Neonatal findings

Fetal–maternal hemorrhage is not a stranger to the brain-damaged neonate. This clinical condition can be confirmed with a maternal KB or similar test. Prior work by Kirkendall and associates [41] demonstrated a relationship between anemic fetuses who had a persistent nonreactive FHR pattern or a placental abruption. Although the KB test results may not be immediately available, the information may provide evidence in selected cases that the fetal–maternal hemorrhage may have antedated maternal admission to the hospital. In the circumstance of a persistent nonreactive FHR pattern, the clinician should attempt to draw the KB test before delivery to potentially avoid contamination caused by the passage of fetal debris into the maternal circulation with delivery [42].

Fetal movement characteristics at the time of maternal admission to the hospital can also provide information as to the timing of fetal brain damage

[43]. The typical fetus who has decreased fetal movement is probably healthy and is usually neurologically normal. At times, the reduced fetal movement can be linked to oligohydramnios [44]. At other times the reduction of fetal movement in association with a persistent nonreactive FHR pattern is significantly more likely to be associated with a fetus who has preadmission impairment [2,12,44]. The documentation of fetal movement characteristics on admission is helpful information not only for timing fetal brain injury but also for providing an explanation to the family of what happened to the fetus.

Umbilical cord blood data can be obtained at the time of birth or later in the nursery. Umbilical cord blood data is not limited to umbilical artery cord blood gases. The clinical focus is on the underlying pathophysiology within the fetal compartment. As implied in Table 1, a complete blood count should be obtained to determine NRBCs and platelets and a chemistry panel to include liver and cardiac enzymes, renal studies, and electrolytes. All of these neonatal parameters have been linked to the intrapartum FHR pattern and the timing of fetal brain injury. For more details on these neonatal blood studies, the reader is referred to the article by Phelan and associates [3]. Finally, abnormalities obtained at or around the time of birth, such as NRBC and serum sodium levels, should be followed frequently in the nursery to document the NRBC clearance or disappearance times and the nadir of the serum sodium.

Placental pathology is an important piece of the fetal brain injury puzzle. The importance is preserving the placenta for histopathologic analysis. When the placenta is analyzed, the pathologist should take cuts in the center of the placenta and where the umbilical cord inserts. Additional cuts should be made in the umbilical cord and any knots in the umbilical cord and any grossly evident abnormality on the fetal or maternal surfaces or umbilical cord. This procedure should be addressed in a meeting between the obstetrics and gynecology department and the chairman or the chairman's representative of the department of pathology. This collaboration permits uniform sectioning of placental and umbilical cord specimens. In the event the department pathologists have limited experience with perinatal pathology, the preserved sections can be forwarded to a pathologist who has specialized training or experience in perinatal pathology.

Finally, video documentation of neonatal or placental findings with a digital camera can permit a visual perspective on the actual clinical findings observed at the time of delivery. As many hospital records are now computer based, the digital images can be uplinked to the patient's medical records for future reference.

Summary

The use of causation and the concept of foreseeability of harm in obstetric malpractice lawsuits have been explored with several fetal brain injury cases and uterine rupture. The application of two approaches, NEC and

Childbirth, to time fetal brain injury were highlighted to underscore their importance as methods to time fetal brain injury. The cornerstone of these methods is that the health care team must become CSIs and gather evidence in cases of a depressed newborn. To assist the health care team a checklist of scientific evidence to be gathered at the time of delivery was provided.

References

[1] Phelan JP. Medico-legal implication of the diagnosis of preeclampsia. In: Belfort MAV, Lyall F, editors. Preeclampsia-aetiology and clinical practice. Boston: Cambridge University Press, in press.

[2] Phelan JP. Perinatal risk management: obstetric methods to prevent birth asphyxia. Clin Perinatol 2005;32:1–17.

[3] Phelan JP, Martin GI, Korst LM. Birth asphyxia and cerebral palsy. Clin Perinatol 2005;32: 61–76.

[4] Brennan TA, Sox CM, Burstin HR. Relation between negligent adverse events and the outcomes of medical-malpractice litigation. N Engl J Med 1996;335:1963–7.

[5] MacPherson v Buick Motor Company, 217 N.Y. 382, 111 N.E. 1050 (1916).

[6] Franklin MA, Rabin RL. Tort law and alternatives: cases and materials. 3rd edition. Mineola (NY): The Foundation Press; 1983.

[7] Rodriguez MH, Masaki DI, Phelan JP, et al. Uterine rupture: are intrauterine pressure catheters useful in the diagnosis? Am J Obstet Gynecol 1989;161:666–9.

[8] Torfs C, Van den Berg BJ, Oeschsli FW, et al. Prenatal and perinatal factors in etiology of cerebral palsy. J Pediatr 1990;116:615–9.

[9] Smith J, Wells L, Dodd K. The continuing fall in incidence of hypoxic-ischaemic encephalopathy in term infants. Br J Obstet Gynecol 2000;107:461–6.

[10] Blair E, Stanley FJ. Intrapartum asphyxia: a rare cause of cerebral palsy. J Pediatr 1988;112: 515–9.

[11] Neonatal Encephalopathy Committee Opinion-2003: American College of Obstetricians and Gynecologists and The American Academy of Pediatrics. Washington, DC.

[12] Phelan JP, Kim JO. Fetal heart rate observations in the brain-damaged infant. Semin Perinatol 2000;24:221–9.

[13] American College of Obstetricians and Gynecologists. Fetal and Neonatal Neurologic Injury. Technical Bulletin No. 163. Washington, DC: American College of Obstetricians and Gynecologists; 1992.

[14] MacLennan A. A template for defining a causal relation between acute intrapartum events and cerebral palsy. BMJ 1999;319:1054–9.

[15] Phelan JP, Ahn MO. Fetal heart rate observations in 300 term brain-damaged infants. J Matern Fetal Investig 1998;8:1–5.

[16] Yeh SY, Diaz F, Paul RH. Ten year experience intrapartum fetal monitoring in Los Angeles County/University of Southern California Medical Center. Am J Obstet Gynecol 1982;143: 496–500.

[17] Perkins RP. Perspectives on perinatal brain damage. Obstet Gynecol 1987;69:807–19.

[18] Phelan JP, Ahn MO. Perinatal observations in forty-eight neurologically impaired term infants. Am J Obstet Gynecol 1994;171:424–31.

[19] Phelan JP. Labor admission test. Clin Perinatol 1994;21(4):879–85.

[20] Ahn MO, Korst LM, Phelan JP. Normal fetal heart rate patterns in the brain-damaged infant: a failure of intrapartum fetal monitoring? J Matern Fetal Investig 1998;8:58–60.

[21] Krebs HB, Petres RE, Dunn LJ. Intrapartum fetal heart rate monitoring VII. Atypical variable decelerations. Am J Obstet Gynecol 1983;145:297–305.

[22] Gaziano EP, Freeman DW. Analysis of heart rate patterns preceding fetal death. Obstet Gynecol 1977;153:721–7.

[23] Electronic fetal heart rate monitoring: research guidelines for interpretation. National Institutes of Child Health and Human Development Research Planning Workshop. Am J Obstet Gynecol 1997;177:1385–8.

[24] Kirkendall C, Phelan JP. Severe acidosis at birth and normal neurologic outcome. Prenat Neonatal Med 2001;6:267–70.

[25] Volpe JJ. Neurology of the newborn. 4th edition. Philadelphia: W.B. Saunders Company; 2001. p. 288.

[26] Low JA, Lindsay BG, Derrick EJ. Threshold of metabolic acidosis associated with newborn complications. Am J Obstet Gynecol 1997;177:1391–4.

[27] Phelan JP, Kirkendall C, Martin G, et al. Neonatal neuroimaging and intrapartum FHR patterns in fetal brain injury. Am J Obstet Gynecol 2001;185(6):S94.

[28] Pasternak JF, Gorey MT. The syndrome of acute near-total intrauterine asphyxia in the term infant. Pediatr Neurol 1998;18:391–8.

[29] Phelan JP, Korst LM, Martin GI. Syndrome of inappropriate antidiuretic hormone (SIADH) among asphyxiated neonates with permanent brain injury: a potential marker to time fetal brain injury. Am J Obstet Gynecol 2006;195:S180.

[30] Phelan JP, Korst LM, Martin GI. Syndrome of inappropriate antidiuretic hormone (SIADH) among asphyxiated neonates with permanent brain injury: the role of intrafetal shunting. Am J Obstet Gynecol 2006;195:S180.

[31] Phelan JP, Korst LM, Martin GI. Validation of the neonatal encephalopathy committee opinion in acutely asphyxiated neonates with permanent brain injury. Am J Obstet Gynecol 2006;195:S22.

[32] Phelan JP, Kirkendall C, Korst L, et al. In cases of fetal brain injury, a slow heart rate at birth is an indicator of severe acidosis. Am J Obstet Gynecol 2003;189(6):S184.

[33] Hon E. An atlas of fetal heart rate patterns. New Haven (CT): Marty Press; 1968.

[34] Krebs HB, Petres RE, Dunn LJ, et al. Intrapartum fetal heart rate monitoring I. Classification and prognosis of fetal heart rate patterns. Am J Obstet Gynecol 1979;133:762.

[35] Greenberg J, Economy K, Mark A, et al. In search of "true" birth asphyxia: labor characteristics associated with the term infant. Am J Obstet Gynecol 2001;185:S94.

[36] Rutherford SE, Phelan JP, Smith CV, et al. The four quadrant assessment of amniotic fluid volume: an adjunct to antepartum fetal heart rate testing. Obstet Gynecol 1987;70:353–6.

[37] Taylor DR, Doughty AS, Kaufman H, et al. Uterine rupture with the use of PGE2 vaginal inserts for labor induction in women with previous cesarean sections. J Reprod Med 2002;47:549–54.

[38] Phelan JP. Uterine rupture. In: Leveno KJ, editor. Obstetric emergencies. Clin Obstet Gynecol 1990;33(3):432–7.

[39] Phelan JP, Korst LM, Settles DK. Uterine activity patterns in uterine rupture: a case–control study. Obstet Gynecol 1998;92:394–7.

[40] Jauregui I, Kirkendall C, Ahn MO, et al. Uterine rupture: a placentally mediated event? Obstet Gynecol 2000;95:75S.

[41] Kirkendall C, Romo M, Phelan JP. FetoMaternal hemorrhage in fetal brain injury. Am J Obstet Gynecol 2001;185(6):S153.

[42] Clark SL, Horenstein J, Phelan JP. Squamous cells in the maternal pulmonary circulation. Am J Obstet Gynecol 1986;154:104–6.

[43] Kirkendall C, Phelan JP. Admission fetal movement characteristics in cases of fetal brain injury. Obstet Gynecol 2002;99(4):47S.

[44] Ahn MO, Phelan JP, Smith CV, et al. Antepartum fetal surveillance in the patient with decreased fetal movement. Am J Obstet Gynecol 1987;157:860–4.

ELSEVIER
SAUNDERS

CLINICS IN
PERINATOLOGY

Clin Perinatol 34 (2007) 439–449

Neonatal Aspects of the Relationship Between Intrapartum Events and Cerebral Palsy

Orna Flidel-Rimon, MD[a,b,*],
Eric Stuart Shinwell, MD[a,b]

[a]Department of Neonatology, Kaplan Medical Center, 76100, Rehovot, Israel
[b]Hebrew University, Jerusalem, Israel

Recent years have witnessed an international, multisource effort to define and progressively improve evidence-based criteria for defining the relationship between perinatal events and the subsequent development of cerebral palsy (CP). In 1992, the American College of Obstetricians and Gynecologists (ACOG) established four basic criteria including umbilical pH less than 7.00, 5-minute Apgar score less than 3, neonatal neurologic sequelae, and multiorgan system dysfunction [1]. Korst and colleagues [2] challenged these criteria by demonstrating that among neonates with an acute catastrophic event characterized by a sudden prolonged fetal heart rate deceleration that lasted until delivery, only 10% of the neonates demonstrated all four of the above criteria. Later, MacLennan [3] defined a template for defining causal relation between acute intrapartum events and cerebral palsy that was developed by the International Cerebral Palsy Task Force after a lengthy and difficult consultative process involving numerous experts. This template, while offering objective criteria, pointed to unresolved issues such as the ability of neuroimaging to determine the timing of an insult, understanding the pathophysiology of the perinatal insult, and the confused terminology used to describe the events. The template included three essential criteria and five nonessential criteria. Subsequently, ACOG [4] has added a fourth essential criterion to the above template and these are now recognized as the current medico-legal standard. Thus, the criteria for defining an acute intrapartum hypoxic event as causal for cerebral palsy include four essential criteria, together with nonspecific criteria that collectively suggest intrapartum timing.

* Corresponding author. Department of Neonatology, Kaplan Medical Center, P.O. Box 1, Rehovot, Israel.
  E-mail address: orna_f@clalit.org.il (O. Flidel-Rimon).

0095-5108/07/$ - see front matter © 2007 Elsevier Inc. All rights reserved.
doi:10.1016/j.clp.2007.06.001
perinatology.theclinics.com

The neonatal components of these criteria include neonatal encephalopathy, Apgar score, multisystem organ dysfunction, and currently available neuroimaging methods. This review will focus on current knowledge and unresolved issues regarding these criteria.

Neonatal encephalopathy

Neonatal encephalopathy (NE) is an all-encompassing term that includes specific conditions such as hypoxic-ischemic encephalopathy secondary to birth asphyxia; however, it is frequently difficult clinically to define a specific cause and effect. MacLennan [3] chose to use the term neonatal encephalopathy rather than hypoxic ischemic encephalopathy, as hypoxia and ischemia in many cases cannot be proven and are assumed from a variety of clinical markers that do not accurately reflect hypoxia and ischemia. NE is a clinically defined syndrome of disturbed neurologic function in the earliest days of life, manifested by difficulties with initiating and maintaining respiration, depression of tone and reflexes, subnormal level of consciousness, and often seizures [5]. Causes of NE include prepartum or postpartum ischemia and hypoxia, genetic factors, metabolic diseases, and maternal drug use. The relative importance of antepartum, intrapartum, and postnatal insults in the pathogenesis of NE is often difficult to quantitate conclusively. Volpe [6] offered approximate percentages based on his own experience and reports of others, showing that primary antepartum insults account for approximately 20% of cases, intrapartum 35%, combined antepartum-intrapartum an additional 35%, and finally 10% are primarily postnatal insults.

The reported incidence of conditions labeled as birth or perinatal asphyxia in term or near-term infants is 1 to 8 neonates per 1000 live term birth and 0.5 to 1.6 per 1000 subsequently developed NE. Of them, between 10% and 60% will die and approximately 25% of the survivors will have long-term neuro-developmental sequelae [7].

The brain can be deprived of oxygen either by hypoxia or ischemia. The principal pathogenic mechanism in intrapartum insults is ischemia secondary to interruption in placental blood flow and gas exchange. Following the initial insult, systemic and cerebral circulatory responses contribute to cerebral reperfusion. Experimental studies have demonstrated that the primary phase of energy failure during the hypoxic ischemic insult in which the brain injury starts is followed by a latent phase of reperfusion during which oxidative metabolism normalizes. The period of reperfusion has been shown to be the time of occurrence of additional deleterious consequences of ischemia on brain metabolism and structure. The acute initial injury tends to result in necrosis, while secondary energy failure after reperfusion tends to lead to apoptotic programmed cell death, with cell shrinkage, karyorhexis, and DNA degradation by specific endonucleases [6,8–10].

Factors that modulate cerebral blood flow during asphyxia include oxygen tension, hypercarbia, and acidosis. The cerebrovascular response (autoregulation) is most marked in the brain stem structures and least in the cerebral white matter. The normal mechanism of autoregulation may be disrupted by hypoxia, hypo- or hypercarbia, or acidosis, causing the cerebral circulation to become pressure-passive and follow the changes in systemic blood pressure. The circulatory response initially includes redistribution of cardiac output to the brain, myocardium, and adrenal at the expense of the kidneys, intestine, and muscle until eventually the decrease in cardiac output is followed by hypotension and decreased cerebral blood flow. The consequence for the brain may be devastating, although the critical threshold for neuronal damage in the developing brain is unknown.

Several systems have been developed to describe the severity of NE and to predict the resulting prognosis (Sarnat, Lipper postasphyxial index, Miller) and, of these, the Sarnat score is the most widely accepted [11]. The staging provides a systematic clinical approach to the identification of those transient neurological signs that appear sequentially following asphyxia near or at the time of birth. The stages correlate with prognosis and also are useful in identifying patients suitable for therapeutic interventions. Three clinical stages of encephalopathy are described.

1. *Stage 1* is characterized by hyperalertness and sympathetic activation, with excessive reaction to stimuli, weak suck with normal tone along with wide-open eyes, decreased blinking, and mydriasis. The electroencephalogram (EEG) is normal during waking. Usually this stage lasts less than 24 hours and is associated with a favorable neurologic outcome.

2. *Stage 2* is characterized by obtundation, hypotonia, strong distal flexion, parasympathetic activation with miosis, slowed heart rate, increased peristalsis and secretions, multifocal seizures, and apneic spells. The EEG shows early relatively low voltage delta and theta wave activity during waking, but isopotential activity persists during sleep. Focal motor seizures are characterized by 1- to 1.5-Hz sharp and slow wave complexes of one hemisphere (usually central or temporal region). The focus may flit between the hemispheres. Stage 2 may last 2 to 14 days.

3. *Stage 3* is characterized with stupor or coma, response to only intense stimulation, with withdrawal or decerebrate posturing and severe hypotonia. Clinical seizures are less frequent than in stage 2. There is a generalized either sympathetic or parasympathetic autonomic dysfunction. Abnormal or absent respiration is noted and the pupils are small or in midposition and poorly react to light. In the EEG, deepened periodic pattern with increased amplitude and decreased frequency of bursts (every 6 to 12 seconds) with further worsening of the picture leading to a very low voltage or isoelectric EEG.

Infants who did not enter stage 3 and who had signs of stage 2 for less than 5 days appeared normal in later infancy. Persistence of stage 2 for more than 7 days or failure of the EEG to revert to normal is frequently associated with later neurologic impairment or death.

The early assessment of the prognosis after NE is important for clinical management. Several studies have confirmed that EEG, when performed within a few days of the hypoxic insult, predicts neurologic outcome accurately. Amplitude-integrated EEG (aEEG) recorded with a cerebral function monitor (CFM) is a single-channel signal obtained from biparietal electrodes. Frequencies less than 2 Hz and more than 15 Hz are filtered selectively and the amplitude-integrated signal is recorded. Studies have shown that the aEEG correlates well with standard EEG, the neurologic outcome, and MRI imaging [12].

Management of infants with NE requires attention to multiple systems including pulmonary, cardiovascular, hepatic, renal, and endocrine function. The emphasis is on prevention of additional hypoxia or ischemia, maintenance of adequate ventilation, perfusion, blood glucose levels, and treatment of seizures.

No specific treatment is yet approved for prevention of neurologic sequelae after NE. However, the fact that there is neuronal loss that occurs during the reperfusion phase led investigators to believe that there may be a therapeutic window in the time period following the initial resuscitation when apoptosis may be aborted or minimized. The most promising intervention is systemic or head cooling, resulting in moderate hypothermia to approximately 34°C. This reduces the cerebral metabolic rate thereby decreasing release of excitatory amino acids, improving the impaired uptake of glutamate, decreasing production of toxic free radicals and NO and preventing apoptotic cell death. Recently, two large multicenter randomized controlled trials have studied the neuro-protective effect of hypothermia. The first study of whole body cooling included infants with a gestational age of at least 36 weeks who had moderate to severe encephalopathy. They were randomly assigned to usual care (control group) or whole body cooling to an esophageal temperature of 33.5°C for 72 hours followed by slow rewarming. The primary outcome was a combined end point of death or moderate to severe disability. There were no adverse effects in the study group and death or severe outcome was seen in 45 of 106 infants in the study group compared with 64 of 103 infants in the control group (relative risk 0.65; 95% confidence interval [CI] 0.44–1.05; $P = .08$). The rate of cerebral palsy was 15 of 77 infants in the study group compared with 19 of 64 infants in the control group (relative risk 0.68; 95% CI 0.38–1.22; $P = .2$). Their conclusions were that whole body hypothermia reduces the risk of death or disability in infants with moderate to severe hypoxic ischemic encephalopathy [13]. In the second study, term infants with moderate to severe NE and abnormal aEEG were randomly assigned to either head cooling for 72 hours within 6 hours of birth with rectal temperature maintained at 34 to 35°C or conventional care. The primary outcome was as above. In the control group, 73 of 110 infants and in the study group 59 of 110 infants died or had severe disability at 18 months (odds ratio 0.66; 95% CI 0.34–1.09; $P = .1$). After adjustment for the severity of the aEEG with logistic regression, the subgroup of moderate NE appeared to benefit most from head cooling. Their conclusions were that the data suggest that while head cooling is not protective in mixed populations of infants with NE, it may safely improve survival without severe neuro-developmental outcome in infants with less-severe aEEG [14]. Although promising, currently further studies are needed to identify the most appropriate target population, the optimal temperature, and the duration of hypothermia.

In summary, the presence of NE is critical in defining the relationship between perinatal insults and subsequent neurological injury [6].

Apgar score

Dr Virginia Apgar [15] proposed in 1952 a quick method for assessing the state of the newborn infant. The score was not originally intended to serve as a predictor of long-term disability, and accordingly its value in predicting outcome has been questioned. The Apgar score is composed of five components—heart rate, respiratory effort, tone, reflex irritability, and color—each of which can be given a score of 0 to 2 for a total of 10. An Apgar score between 7 and 10 is considered normal. The score have many limitations. For example, each of the five factors that make up the score is given equal weight, and clearly the importance of each for central nervous system integrity is not equal. Factors that may affect the accuracy of the score include drugs, trauma, congenital anomalies, infections, prematurity, hypovolemia, and hypoxia. The Apgar score has a limited time frame. It was shown by Clark and Hakanson [16] that when groups of health care providers were compared there was interobserver inconsistency. After showing videos of resuscitations, interobserver agreement was seen in 68% of pediatricians and pediatric house staff, 46% of obstetricians and obstetric house staff, and 42% of intensive care nursery staff, while obstetric nurses and community hospital nurses had even lower rates.

A national cohort study in Norway from 1983 to 1987 assessed the relationship between low Apgar scores and adverse neurologic outcome. The study included 235,165 children with birth weight of at least 2500 g who did not have birth defects. The children were followed until age 8 to 12 years. Infants who had 5-minute Apgar score of 0 to 3 had a 386-fold increase in neonatal death, a 76-fold increase in death during the first year of life, and an 81-fold increase in cerebral palsy as compared with infants who had scores of 7 to 10 at age 5 minutes [17]. A similar study was performed by Casey and colleagues [18] on 132,228 term infants. The mortality rate was 244 of 1000 live births with Apgar score of 0 to 3, and only 0.2 of 1000 when the score was 7 to 10 at age 5 minutes. They also showed that the 5-minute Apgar score was a better predictor than umbilical-artery pH, although the combination of 5-minute Apgar score of 0 to 3 together with umbilical-artery pH less than 7.00 significantly increased the relative risk of death in neonates. This study was limited by the relatively small number of infants with very low 5-minute Apgar score—only 178 of 145,624 preterm and term infants. However, it is important to keep in mind that the use of the Apgar score to define birth asphyxia is essentially a misapplication. The American Academy of Pediatrics (AAP), together with ACOG, issued a statement regarding the Apgar score in 1986 and have since revised it twice most recently in 2006 [19–21]. The main messages are the following:

1. Apgar score describes the condition of the newborn infant after birth. The change in the score between 1 and 5 minutes is a useful index of the response to resuscitation.
2. Low 1-minute score alone does not correlate with future outcome. Apgar score of 0 to 3 at 5 minutes may correlate with neonatal mortality, but alone does not predict later neurologic dysfunction. Low Apgar score in combination with other markers of asphyxia may identify infants at risk of developing seizures. The risk of poor neurologic outcomes increases when Apgar score is 3 or less at 10, 15, and 20 minutes.

Multiple organ involvement

Multisystem organ dysfunction was considered in the past as a clinical requirement to support the claim that a neonate had been asphyxiated. In the current task force, it is a nonspecific criterion that together with other criteria may suggest intrapartum timing of an insult. Multisystem organ dysfunction is mechanistically related to the diving reflex. Following asphyxia, there is shunting of blood from the skin and splanchnic area to the heart, adrenal, and brain to protect these vital organs. Thus, it is likely that severe asphyxia will be followed by dysfunction of other organs that are less essential, such as the kidneys, liver, and gut. Shunting of blood through the ductus venosus will cause subsequent hepatic hypoxia with elevation of liver enzymes. Ischemia and hypoxia can cause renal damage resulting in decreased renal function and acute tubular necrosis with oliguria, hematuria, and proteinuria.

The relative significance of multisystem injury in the establishment of a causal relationship between acute intrapartum events and cerebral palsy has been studied. Hankins and colleagues [22] examined the proportion of major organ systems injured in 46 cases of acute peripartum asphyxia that resulted in NE. They found that elevated liver enzymes occurred in 80%, heart injury (defined by need for pressors or volume support beyond 2 hours of life) occurred in 78%, and renal injury (defined by increased creatinine, proteinuria, hematuria, or clinical oliguria) occurred in 72% of the cases. They concluded that evidence of multiple organ system damage was the rule with cases that clearly demonstrated acute intrapartum asphyxia that resulted in neonatal encephalopathy. In 67% of patients, the pH was less than 7.00, and in 83% of the patients 5-minute Apgar score was less than 6. In a later correspondence they reported that among the 46 infants with NE, all had at least one other organ system injury beyond that of the central nervous system [23].

To evaluate their suitability for organ transplantation, the pathology of the kidneys, lungs, liver, and intestine was assessed in 35 infants who died of postasphyxia NE. Severe pathological changes were observed in the following proportion of cases: heart, 62%; lungs, 33%%; kidneys, 28%; liver, 22%; and gut, 6%. In 9 of 35, two or more organs were found. The proportion of organs with no pathological changes included heart, 17%; lungs, 0%; kidneys, 14%; and liver, 14%. Barnett and colleagues also found that matching of clinical and pathological categories of severity was imperfect [24]. Another study from the same center assessed the pattern of involvement of each major system and showed that all infants with HIE had evidence for at least one organ dysfunction [25]. Somewhat different results were seen in another study in which no additional organ system dysfunction was seen in 14 (36%) of 57 cases that had hypoxic ischemic encephalopathy (HIE) with permanent neurologic injury [26]. All 57 cases were later diagnosed with cerebral palsy. This suggests that acute fetal neurologic injury can happen so quickly that there may not be sufficient time for shunting of blood to occur. Thus, the absence of organ dysfunction should be considered, in selected circumstances, with an acute fetal neurologic insult.

The available imaging methods

Neuroimaging in infants with NE plays an important role in diagnosis and provides prognostic information regarding risk for long-term neurodevelopmental disability. In addition, neuroimaging may be helpful in evaluating the exact time of the insult.

Clinical examination of term infants with signs and symptoms of NE often cannot determine the severity of the cerebral damage and provides little information regarding the etiology of the insult. The American Academy of Neurology (AAN) has published a practice parameter for neuroimaging of the neonate [27]. Their recommendations for diagnostic assessment are the following:

1. For infants with history of neonatal encephalopathy, significant birth trauma, and evidence for low hematocrit or coagulopathy, a noncontrast CT should be performed to look for hemorrhage and if the CT finding cannot explain the clinical status of the neonate, MRI should be performed.
2. For other neonates with acute encephalopathy, MRI should be performed between days 2 and 8 of life. In addition, if single-voxel magnetic resonance spectrometry (MRS) is available, MRI should include MRS. At the time of MRI, DWI (diffusion weighted imaging) should also be performed if this modality is available. CT should be performed only if MRI is not available or if the neonate is too unstable for MRI.

The major neuropathological varieties of HIE include the following basic subtypes [6,8].

Selective neural necrosis

Selective neural necrosis is the most common injury observed, including necrosis of neurons in widespread distribution, associated with severe and prolonged insult, seen in both preterm and term infants. Cerebral cortical-deep nucleus involvement is associated with prolonged moderate to severe insult usually in term infants, often associated with involvement of the basal ganglia and thalamus. Deep nuclear and brain stem involvement is predominantly in term infants after severe but abrupt insults. Pontosubicular injury (type of selective neuronal injury with involvement of the basis pontis, and the subiculum of hippocampus) is more common in preterm infants. The long-term sequelae include mental retardation and seizures.

Parasagittal cerebral injury

Parasagittal cerebral injury refers to a lesion of the cerebral cortex and subcortical white matter with a characteristic distribution. It is characterized by bilateral necrosis of the cortex and adjacent subcortical white matter, involving mainly the posterior, but also superior and medial aspects of the cerebral convexities. This is characteristic of the term infant with perinatal asphyxia. The areas of necrosis are in the border zones between the fields of major cerebral arteries, which are susceptible to a fall in cerebral perfusion pressure. The most frequent of long-term sequelae is spastic quadriplegia.

Periventricular leukomalacia

Periventricular leukomalacia refers to necrosis of white matter in a characteristic distribution, in the white matter dorsal and lateral to the external angles of the lateral ventricles. It is the principal ischemic lesion of the preterm infant. The long-term manifestations include spastic diplegia and spastic quadriplegia, with visual and cognitive deficits in severe injury [28].

Focal and multifocal ischemic brain necrosis

Focal and multifocal ischemic brain necrosis is characterized by injury to all cellular elements caused by infarction within a vascular distribution. Involvement of the middle cerebral artery occurred in one half of the cases. Later it will present as porencephaly, multicystic encephalomalacia, and hydraencephaly. The long-term neurologic sequelae are related to the location and extent of the primary lesion and include spastic hemiplegia, spastic quadriplegia, and seizures [6].

The most appropriate neuroimaging modality varies according to the suspected condition. Cranial ultrasound is noninvasive, portable, and widely available and is the best tool for identification of periventricular leukomalacia. It is also useful in the identification of injury to the basal ganglia and thalamus and focal and multifocal ischemic brain injury. In a study of early cranial ultrasound changes in 70 healthy term infants with 104 asphyxiated infants, abnormal changes were seen in a significantly higher proportion of asphyxiated infants, but those changes were not predictors of adverse outcome during the first year of life [29]. The AAN concluded that here are little data to support the use of ultrasound in imaging of the encephalopathic term infant [27].

CT scan may provide important diagnostic information in identification of diffuse cortical injury in severe selective neuronal necrosis, injury to basal ganglia and thalamus, and focal and multifocal ischemic brain necrosis. It is limited in the identification of parasagittal cerebral injury and venous thrombosis, and also only moderately useful for identification of periventricular leukomalacia. CT scan changes are shown by 24 hours after injury.

The AAN concluded that CT can detect low attenuation in the basal ganglia and thalami indicating severe injury that is consistent with HIE. Other studies demonstrated that CT plays a role in detecting hemorrhagic lesions [27].

MRI is the most informative imaging modality. Unfortunately, MRI is not always available and sometimes the infants are too unstable for this procedure. Standard MRI sequences show absence of the normal high T1 in the posterior limb of the internal capsule by about 24 hours. Rutherford and colleagues [30] showed that abnormal signal intensity in the posterior limb of the internal capsule (PLIC) is an accurate early predictor of poor outcome in infants with HIE. In 36 of 73 infants with HIE who had abnormal signal intensity, 16 died and 20 had a developmental delay at the age of 1 year, while 32 of the 73 had normal signal, 28 normal outcome (3 had mild developmental delay and 1 died), and equivocal signal intensity was seen in 5 infants. Abnormal high signal appears in the lateral thalami and posterior lentiform nuclei by the third day of life. This high signal becomes a smaller focus in the lateral thalamus and posterior putamen and remains visible for 2 to 4 months. High T2 signal appears in this area by the end of the second week [29].

Volpe [6] stated that MRI is the diagnostic modality of choice in the immediate neonatal period in infants with HIE. The entire spectrum of hypoxic ischemic brain has been demonstrated [4]. The AAN concluded that characteristic MR patterns of cerebral injury can be detected using conventional T1- to T2-weighted imaging sequences performed at mean ages of 2 to 8 days [27]. Diffusion-weighted MRI (DWI), based on the molecular diffusion of water, is more sensitive than conventional MRI, and shows abnormalities earlier, from first hour after birth [31,32].

The pattern of injury after hypoxic ischemic event depends on the gestational age of the infant and on the duration and severity of the insult to the brain. MRI is the best diagnostic and prognostic modality. It has shown that there are characteristic HIE-associated lesions, and these have been shown to correlate with the type of hypoxic ischemic insult. The abnormalities may be obvious within few days after delivery. Neuroimaging, mainly MRI, is an important tool in helping to define the cause of neonatal encephalopathy and also the approximate time of the insult.

Summary

We have reviewed the value and limitations of NE, Apgar score, multisystem dysfunction, and neuroimaging in the relationship between intrapartum events and neurologic outcome. Critical appraisal of these findings allows acceptable accuracy in confirming or refuting a causal relationship in most cases.

References

[1] The American college of obstetricians and gynecologists. Fetal and neonatal neurologic injury. Technical Bulletin# 163. Washington, DC: American College of Obstetricians and gynecologists; 1992.

[2] Korst LM, Phelan JP, Wang YM, et al. Acute fetal asphyxia and permanent brain injury: a retrospective analysis of current indicators. J Matern Fetal Med 1999;8:101–6.

[3] MacLennan A. A template for defining a causal relation between acute intrapartum events and cerebral palsy: international consensus statement. BMJ 1999;319:1054–9.

[4] The American College of Obstetricians and Gynecologists, task force on neonatal encephalopathy and cerebral palsy; American Academy of Pediatrics. Neonatal encephalopathy and cerebral palsy: defining the pathogenesis and pathophysiology. Washington, DC: American College of Obstetricians and Gynecologists; 2003.

[5] Leviton A, Nelson KB. Neonatal encephalopathy: problems with definitions and classifications. Paediatr Neurol 1992;8:85–90.

[6] Volpe JJ. Neurology of the newborn. 4th edition. Philadelphia: W.B. Saunders company; 2001. p. 217–331.

[7] Badawi N, Kurinczuk JJ, Keogh JM, et al. Intrapartum risk factors for newborn encephalopathy: the western Australian case-control study. BMJ 1998;317:1554–8.

[8] Perlman JM. Intrapartum hypoxic-ischemic cerebral injury and subsequent cerebral palsy: medicolegal issues. Pediatrics 1997;99:851–9.

[9] Lorek A, Takei Y, Cady EB, et al. Delayed ("secondary") cerebral energy failure after acute hypoxia-ischemia in the newborn piglet: continuous 48 hour studies by phosphorus magnetic resonance spectroscopy. Pediatr Res 1994;36:699–706.

[10] Levene MI, Chervenak FA, Whittle MJ, et al, editors. Fetal and neonatal neurology and neurosurgery. 3rd edition. Churchill Livingstone; 2001. p. 323–8.

[11] Sarnat HB, Sarnat MS. Neonatal encephalopathy following fetal distress. Arch Neurol 1976; 33:696–705.

[12] Al Naqeeb N, Edwards AD, Cowan FM, Azzopardi D. Assesment of neonatal encephalopathy by amplitude integrated electroencephalography. Pediatrics 1999;103:1263–71.

[13] Shankaran S, Laptook AR, Ehrenkrantz RA, NICHD neonatal research network, et al. Whole-body hypothermia for neonates with hypoxic-ischemic encephalopathy. N Engl J Med 2005;353:1574–84.

[14] Gluckman PD, Wyatt JS, Azzopardi D, et al. Selective head cooling with mild systemic hypothermia after neonatal encephalopathy. Multicentre randomized trial. Lancet 2005; 365:663–70.

[15] Apgar V. A proposal for a new method of evaluation of the newborn infant. Curr Res Anes Anal 1953;32:260–7.

[16] Clark D, Hakanson D. The inaccuracy of Apgar scoring. J Perinatol 1988;8:203–5.

[17] Moster D, Lie RT, Irgens LM, et al. The association of Apgar score with subsequent death and cerebral palsy: a population-based study in term infants. J Pediatr 2001;138:798–803.

[18] Casey BM, McIntire DD, Leveno KJ. The continuing value of the Apgar score for the assessment of newborn infants. N Engl J Med 2001;344:467–71.

[19] Committee on fetus and newborn. Use and abuse of the Apgar score. Pediatrics 1986;78: 1148–9.

[20] Committee on fetus and newborn, American Academy of Pediatrics and Committee on obstetric practice, American college of Obstetric and Gynecologosts. Use and abuse of the Apgar score. Pediatrics 1996;98:141–2.

[21] American Academy of Pediatrics, committee on fetus and newborn, American college of Obstetric and Gynecologosts and Committee on obstetric practice. The Apgar score. Pediatrics 2006;117:1444–7.

[22] Hankins GDV, Koen S, Gei AF, et al. Neonatal organ system failure in acute birth asphyxia sufficient to result in neonatal encephalopathy. Obstet Gynecol 2002;99:688–91.

[23] Lam MH. Neonatal organ system failure in acute birth asphyxia sufficient to result in neonatal encephalopathy. Obstet Gynecol 2003;101:203–4 [letter to the editor].

[24] Barnett CP, Perlman M, Ekert PG. Clinicopathological correlation in postasphyxial organ damge: a donor organ perspective. Pediatrics 1997;99:797–9.

[25] Shah P, Riphagen S, Beyene J, et al. Multiorgan dysfunction in infants with post-asphyxial hypoxic-ischemic encephalopathy. Arch Dis Child Fetal Neonatal Ed 2004;89:F152–5.

[26] Phelan JP, Ahn MO, Korst L, et al. Intrapartum fetal asphyxial brain injury with absent multiorgan system dysfunction. J Matern Fetal Med 1998;7:19–22.

[27] Ment LR, Bada HS, Barnes P, et al. Practice parameter: neuroimaging of the neonate. Report of the quality standards subcommittee of the American academy of neurology and the practice committee of the child neurology society. Neurology 2002;58:1726–38.

[28] Perlman JM, Risser R, Broyles RS. Bilateral cystic periventricular leukomalacia in the premature infant: associated risk factors. Pediatrics 1996;97:822–7.

[29] Boo NY, Chandran V, Zulfiqar MA, et al. Early cranial ultrasound changes as predictors of outcome during first year of life in term infants with peripheral asphyxia. J Paediatr Child Health 2000;36:363–9.

[30] Rutherford MA, Pennock JM, Counsell SJ, et al. Abnormal magnetic resonance signal in the internal capsule predicts poor neurodevelopmental outcome in infants with hypoxic ischemic encephalopathy. Pediatrics 1998;102:323–8.

[31] Barkovich AJ, Westmark KD, Ferriero DM, et al. Perinatal asphyxia: MR finding in the first 10 days. AJNR Am J Neuroradiol 1995;16:427–38.

[32] Robertson RL, Ben-Sira L, Barnes PD, et al. MR line scan diffusion imaging of term neonates with perinatal brain ischemia. AJNR Am J Neuroradiol 1999;20:1658–70.

ELSEVIER
SAUNDERS

Clin Perinatol 34 (2007) 451–459

CLINICS IN
PERINATOLOGY

Umbilical Cord Blood Gases

Isaac Blickstein, MD[a,b,*], Tamar Green, MD[a]

[a]*Department of Obstetrics and Gynecology, Kaplan Medical Center, 76100 Rehovot, Israel*
[b]*Hadassah-Hebrew University School of Medicine, Jerusalem, Israel*

The intrapartum acid-base status of the fetus is an important component in establishing the link between intrapartum events and neonatal condition. Because all methods for assessing the acid-base condition during labor (such as fetal heart rate tracing and direct pH assessment from the fetal scalp) have a disappointingly low predictive power, umbilical cord blood gas levels are believed to be the best representation of the fetal acid-base status immediately before birth.

When an adverse neonatal condition is alleged to be related to an intrapartum hypoxic event, it is logical to assume that the cord blood gases will show significant acidemia. This logical assumption is corroborated by numerous data that relate cord blood acidemia to the subsequent development of cerebral palsy (CP). In simplistic terms, when the oxygen supply to the fetus is significantly disrupted, tissue oxygen deprivation develops, acids begin to accumulate, and acidemia ensues.

Because cord blood gases can be objectively measured and because they accurately represent the fetal condition just before birth, their level is one of the essential criteria used to define an acute intrapartum hypoxic event [1,2]. Using this definition, a normal pH value practically excludes a causal relationship between the intrapartum period and subsequent development of brain damage. Thus, determination of cord blood gases is frequently an important and invaluable argument in litigation. This article discusses various aspects of this measurement.

Development of damaging acidosis

Intrapartum asphyxia, defined as acute interruption of oxygen supply, commonly occurs when the placenta, for one reason or another, is hypoperfused.

---

* Corresponding author.
  E-mail address: blick@netvision.net.il (I. Blickstein).

doi:10.1016/j.clp.2007.05.001

In such a circumstance, retention of carbon dioxide (CO_2) occurs. Because the fetus normally clears CO_2 by way of the placental circulation, the finding of increased partial pressure of CO_2 (PCO_2) in the cord blood analysis is a marker of respiratory acidosis. In contrast to the adult, if the asphyxia is not corrected, metabolic acidosis eventually develops and creates a state of mixed respiratory and metabolic acidosis. Over time, the respiratory component dissipates and, finally, almost pure metabolic acidosis is found.

In all these phases, acidemia is present (ie, a low pH is found in the blood sample). The cutoff value for damaging acidosis is set at pH less than 7.00 because it is unlikely that acute acidosis with pH values greater than 7.00 could be directly associated with CP [1]. Moreover, because respiratory acidosis is of little consequence in terms of outcome, the metabolic component of damaging acidemia is of importance. Hence, the definition used as an essential criterion is pH less than 7.00 and base deficit (bicarbonate [HCO_3]) greater than 12 mmol/L [1,2].

The final pH of blood is determined by the proportion between the PCO_2 (respiratory) component and the HCO_3 (metabolic) component. This construct suggests that when metabolic acidemia is found, the timing of the hypoxic insult cannot be estimated. In contrast, when a respiratory component is found, the onset of hypoxic insult can be established because this component cannot last more than 20 to 30 minutes (usually less). Furthermore, one can establish what the pH was before the acute insult by reducing the respiratory component. This calculation can be performed by the method described by Eisenberg and colleagues [3]. In the first step, one subtracts the value of the normal neonatal PCO_2 (50 mm Hg) from the PCO_2 value found in the blood gas analysis to establish the excess in CO_2. Next, given that every 10 mm Hg of the PCO_2 reduces the pH by 0.08, the excess PCO_2 is divided by 10 and multiplied by 0.08. Finally, the resultant respiratory acidosis component is added to the pH to establish the mixed acidosis level.

For example, an acute hypoxic event occurred during labor and the attending physicians rushed the patient for a prompt cesarean. The baby was delivered within 14 minutes. The claim was that the attending staff overlooked signs of fetal distress before the hypoxic event that prompted the cesarean. Cord blood gases showed a pH of 6.90 and a PCO_2 of 100 mm Hg. Using the previously mentioned calculation, the excess of PCO_2 is $100 - 50 = 50$ mm Hg. The respiratory acidosis level is calculated as $50 \div 10 = 5 \times 0.08 = 0.4$. From this cord gas level, one can deduce that the pH before respiratory acidosis started was $6.90 + 0.4 = 7.30$, a perfectly normal value. Thus, the allegation that a nonreassuring fetal heart rate tracing was present before the acute hypoxic event is very unlikely.

Another example describes a patient admitted to the hospital with a nonreassuring admission fetal heart rate tracing. After some initial observation, the patient was rushed for a prompt cesarean. The claim was that damage occurred after admission. Cord blood gases showed a pH of 6.90 and a PCO_2 of 60 mm Hg. Using the same calculation, the excess of PCO_2 is

$60 - 50 = 10$ mm Hg and the respiratory acidosis level is $10 \div 10 = 1 \times 0.08 = 0.08$, for a pH value of $6.90 + 0.08 = 6.98$, a level considered damaging acidemia. These cord blood gases, uncorrected by a respiratory component, cannot support a recent asphyxia event; in fact, they cannot tell us when the damaging acidemia occurred.

Indication for sampling

Because cord blood gas analysis is a useful proxy for fetal condition just before birth, it would ideally be performed after every delivery, just as an Apgar score is determined. This approach is not practical, however, because in most cases, cord blood gas analysis is not necessary in the vigorous newborn. The recent American College of Obstetricians and Gynecologists committee opinion on umbilical cord gas analysis [4] described the indications for sampling. In general, cord blood sampling for acid-base status is advisable when an intrapartum event might be associated (correctly or not) with an adverse outcome. This admittedly defensive approach might prove critical when the case is under medicolegal dispute and when exclusion of an intrapartum event by demonstrating a normal pH value is needed.

The 1999 consensus statement [1] pointed out that some intrapartum signs that prompt an obstetric intervention "may mistakenly be taken as evidence of acute compromise" in a chronically compromised case. Therefore, prompt instrumental or abdominal delivery for suspected fetal compromise should always be followed by cord blood gas analysis. This indication can be extended to all nonelective cesareans. Similar arguments exist for a low 5-minute Apgar score, an abnormal fetal heart rate tracing, intrauterine growth restriction, intrapartum fever, and multiple pregnancy [4].

As previously noted, all three essential criteria (one criterion being metabolic acidosis with a pH < 7.00) are necessary to establish causation between intrapartum asphyxia and CP. The (medicolegal) question may arise in the absence of this information. In such cases, the consensus maintains that "if blood gas data are not available, it cannot be assumed from other signs that hypoxia was present at birth since these signs lack specificity either individually or as a group" [1].

Given the accepted prevalence of CP of 2 per 1000 normally grown term infants, an obstetric service with 3000 deliveries per year will have 6 CP cases annually [5]. Five of these 6 cases are expected to be delivered without asphyxia. These investigators [5] maintain that with the current medicolegal environment, when settlements for CP are regularly over £3 million, including a full blood gas analysis might prove to be cost-effective in delivery suite budgets.

Sampling the artery alone versus sampling the artery and vein

The umbilical vein carries oxygenated blood to the fetus, whereas the two umbilical arteries carry deoxygenated blood in the opposite direction, from the fetus to the placenta. Thus, arterial blood reflects fetal acid-base balance with a lower pH and P_{CO_2} and a higher P_{CO_2} than venous blood, which reflects a combination of the fetal and the maternal acid-base status. For this reason, it is widely accepted that the umbilical artery provides the most accurate information for detecting fetal or neonatal acid-base status. Consequently, to compare results from different studies, one must identify the vessel that was sampled and, in particular, compare the results to the accepted standard. Admittedly, several investigators did not specify which vessel was sampled; however, most studies referred to arterial pH values and others used venous values because of some difficulty in obtaining samples from the artery.

In Waugh and colleagues' [5] survey of 181 obstetric units in the United Kingdom performing cord blood gas analyses, 98 (54%) sampled arterial and venous blood and 33 (18%) sampled venous blood only. The main reason for sampling both vessels is to be sure to identify the artery. The 26th Royal College of Obstetricians and Gynaecologists' Study Group on Intrapartum Fetal Surveillance [6] also recommended obtaining blood from artery and vein. Westgate and colleagues [7] examined the relationship between blood gases of the umbilical artery and vein and concluded that it is essential to sample both vessels to ensure that separate vessels were sampled. In their analysis, very large arterial–venous differences existed (0.02–0.49 for pH, 0.5–9.9 kPa for P_{CO_2}, and 11.8–9.7 for base excess); therefore, a normal venous pH is unable to exclude the possibility of significant arterial acidosis. Moreover, differences in pH and base excess may provide some information about the time course of acidosis because a large arterial–venous base excess difference may indicate an acute event, whereas a small arterial–venous base excess difference is more likely to indicate a chronic acidosis course [7].

Technical aspects

Blood and the placenta are living organs, and metabolism may continue extracorporeal for some time after delivery. It follows, at least in theory, that if blood is not sampled correctly or immediately, if shipment of the sample is inappropriate, or if assessment is deferred for some reason, then the results of the analysis might become inaccurate because of further metabolism by the blood and the placenta.

Sampling site

A potential confounder of blood sampling—the sampling site—was also evaluated. Nodwell and colleagues [8] measured blood gases, pH, O_2 saturation, and hemoglobin in artery and in vein from the umbilical cord and from the placental cord insertion. They found that partial pressure of oxygen (P_{O_2}) and O_2 saturation were lower in the placental vein compared with the umbilical vein and that P_{CO_2} was lower and pH was higher in the placental artery compared with the umbilical artery. These researchers concluded that placental cord blood provides a close estimation of fetal base excess and hemoglobin status at birth, but with a larger error for Po_2, O_2 saturation, Pco_2, and pH due to continued gas exchange within and across the placenta after cord clamping. Perlman and colleagues [9] showed consistent and significant increases in arterial pH and Pco_2 and a decrease in Po_2 from samples obtained along the umbilical cord, from near the fetal origin to the placental cord insertion. The largest difference was noted between the fetal origin and the placental plate. Perlman and colleagues [9] concluded that the sampling site should be standardized and that the umbilical artery should be sampled at the site nearest to the fetus.

Effect of timing

Controversy exists regarding the best time for sampling the umbilical cord blood. To date, different studies have yielded somewhat different conclusions. Hilger and colleagues [10] studied whether a delay in blood sampling affects the values of placental blood gases, pH, and calculated bicarbonate. Blood was sampled serially at 15, 30, 45, and 60 minutes following delivery of normal term neonates. Placentas and cords were stored at room temperature. When the umbilical vein was sampled, time had no effect, whereas serial samples taken from the placental surface vessels showed a statistically and biologically significant decrease in pH and increase in Pco_2 over time. In contrast, Strickland and coauthors [11] evaluated blood sampling for pH and Pco_2 stored at room temperature for variable intervals after delivery and concluded that blood samples can be left at room temperature for up to 30 minutes without significant affect on these values. Similarly, Duerbeck and colleagues [12] evaluated the effect of delayed sampling from clamped umbilical cord segments. Umbilical artery blood samples were collected in nonheparinized and noniced plastic syringes and processed immediately. No significant changes in the tested blood gas parameters were noted 60 minutes after delivery.

Because determination of acid-base status within 60 minutes of birth is not feasible in all hospitals on a 24-hour basis, Chauhan and colleagues [13] evaluated whether the alternative of performing arterial cord blood gas analysis hours after sampling at birth would still reliably identify the acidotic newborn. Multiple umbilical arterial blood samples were withdrawn into five preheparinized syringes and analyzed at 0.5, 15, 30, 45, and 60 hours after birth. The investigators developed mathematic models that would allow the clinician to identify the acidotic newborn when the time interval from delivery to blood gas analysis and the remote values of pH and base deficit are known. As expected, the remote gas analysis inaccurately identified almost 70% (11/16) of normal newborns as being acidotic at birth. Using the mathematical equations, however, the identification of the acidotic neonate was still possible even after 60 hours post delivery.

More recently, Valenzuela and Guijarro [14] evaluated pH, P_{O_2}, and P_{CO_2} in arterial and venous umbilical vessels drawn 5, 60, and 120 minutes post partum. After 60 minutes, the average values for pH in the arterial–venous paired samples were similar, although P_{CO_2} in both vessels decreased significantly and arterial P_{O_2} increased significantly. After 120 minutes, however, significant changes were noted in the arterial pH (increase) and in arterial and venous P_{CO_2} (decrease). The significant differences that occurred over time, however, were clinically insignificant, suggesting that when immediate analysis of umbilical cord blood gases is impossible, the measurement obtained later could still be useful. These findings did not concur with those of Paerregaard and colleagues [15] who observed more than 25 years ago in a small series of 11 cases that variations in pH and P_{O_2} were modest at 15 minutes but significant at 30 minutes after delivery.

Effect of cord clamping

As discussed earlier, the potential communication of the umbilical vessels with the placenta might confound the acid-base status determination. Thus, isolation of the vessels by clamping the cord might be advisable. Armstrong and Stenson [16] questioned the role of clamping the cord immediately after delivery (to isolate the vessel from the placenta) on the timing for sampling the vessels. These investigators found that arterial and venous lactate was significantly higher by 20 minutes compared with time 0 in clamped and un-clamped vessels and that changes in unclamped vessels were greater than in clamped vessels. The pH remained unchanged after 60 minutes in clamped vessels but changed significantly in unclamped vessels. The base excess changed significantly in clamped and unclamped vessels. These findings led the authors to conclude that delayed sampling from unclamped cords is very unreliable and that cord blood samples taken after 20 minutes are unreliable for lactate measurement. It follows that current guidelines stating that blood can be sampled from a clamped cord for up to 1 hour after delivery should not be applied to the interpretation of lactate or base excess.

Effect of temperature

Low temperature may inhibit biologic processes occurring over time in the blood sample and, theoretically, may allow a longer time interval between sampling cord blood and assessing pH and blood gases. Thus, the discussion regarding the best time for sampling cord blood for pH and gases cannot be separated from the discussion regarding the best temperature for keeping the sample until it reaches the laboratory. In one of the earliest studies on cord blood analyses, Sato and Saling [17] stored blood at room temperature and in a refrigerator. The former was tested for pH every 5 minutes up to 80 minutes, and the pH measurements of the refrigerated blood were performed after 30 minutes and then every hour for up to 7 hours and, finally, after 24 hours. The results of this study suggested that if fetal blood cannot be assessed at less than 50 minutes, it must be kept refrigerated to inhibit auto-oxidation.

Similarly, Strickland and colleagues [11] evaluated blood being sampled for pH and P_{CO_2} that was stored at room temperature for variable intervals after delivery. They concluded that blood samples can be left at room temperature for up to 30 minutes.

Manor and colleagues [18] tested three pairs of blood samples in heparin-containing syringes immediately after delivery, after 1 hour at room temperature, and after 1 hour in a refrigerator. No significant changes were detected in blood gases and pH among the three pairs of samples. These data corroborate those of Sykes and Molloy [19] and indicate that during an interval of 1 hour, temperature does not significantly affect the levels of pH, P_{CO_2}, and P_{O_2}.

Effect of heparin

Heparin is necessary to prevent blood samples from clotting in the syringe or in the analyzer; thus, blood samples are obtained in preheparinized syringes or in syringes flushed with heparin. The problem with heparin, however, is that it is acidic and may introduce error in the pH and P_{CO_2} measurements if its amount exceeds 10% of the volume of any blood sample.

More than 20 years ago, Sykes and Molloy [19] and Pel and Treffers [20] compared samplings that had been left at room temperature and in a refrigerator and found conflicting results that were attributed to differences in the dose of heparin in the collecting syringes. In contrast, Westgate and colleagues [7] did not find significant differences when comparing results from nonheparinized and heparinized syringes. Standardization of the amount of heparin that remains after flushing of the syringes seems advisable, and the accepted method for preheparinization is to add one drop of heparin from a 1-mL tuberculin syringe into a 2-mL plastic syringe, moving the plunger up and down and expelling any residual heparin with a 21-gauge needle.

Summary

Intrapartum signs such as a nonreassuring fetal heart rate or meconium staining of the amniotic fluid may be signs of chronic neurologic compromise [1,2]. These signs may frequently precipitate an obstetric intervention performed in the hope that the pathology is of recent onset and therefore still reversible [1]. The action of the obstetric team in such cases may mistakenly be considered supporting evidence of acute compromise and supporting the allegation that some omission during the intrapartum care led to brain damage of the fetus/neonate. Thus, clear-cut, evidence-based, or consensus-based criteria are needed to exclude the potential association between an intrapartum event and brain damage.

**Box 1. Recommendations of the American College
of Obstetricians and Gynecologists for umbilical
cord blood gas sampling**

- Double clamp an umbilical cord segment immediately after birth.
- Obtain a blood sample with a syringe flushed with heparin.
- A paired sampling of the artery and vein may prevent a dispute over the accuracy of arterial sampling.
- If the neonate appears vigorous, then the clamped cord segment can be discarded.
- The cord segment is appropriate for sampling anytime within 60 minutes from birth.
- Blood is appropriate for analysis anytime within 60 minutes from sampling.

This article discusses various aspects of cord blood gas levels, one of the essential criteria for determining a causal relationship between intrapartum asphyxia and subsequent development of CP. The data presented in this article support the logic behind this criterion because assessment of cord blood gases is an objective and reliable measure of the acid-base status just before birth. In contrast to the more subjective Apgar score (a reliable tool to identify neonates in need of immediate postpartum treatment), the role of blood gas analysis is to complement the Apgar score in elucidating whether that need is a result of an acute antepartum event. Taken together, blood gas analysis should be an integral part of every neonatal assessment when it might be required to establish causation between intrapartum events and adverse outcome.

The assessment of cord blood gases is simple. It takes only a few minutes to complete sampling, measuring, and shipping. Little doubt exists about the accuracy of an appropriate sample (Box 1) [4]. The technical aspects discussed earlier are primarily intended to identify circumstances when a sample may be considered inappropriate and thus inaccurate [4–6]. Most of the studies related to the accuracy of cord blood acid-base status examined extreme situations during the era before automated equipment was commonplace. It appears that in well-equipped and adequately staffed obstetric services, a substantial deviation from the standard procedure is required before a sample is alleged to be imprecise. Moreover, a wide margin of accuracy exists even when prompt assessment is not available because of a busy obstetric service or simply because measurement is not available on a 24-hour basis; hence, it is doubtful whether standard sampling methods would be ineligible in litigation.

References

[1] MacLennan A. A template for defining a causal relation between acute intrapartum events and cerebral palsy: international consensus statement. BMJ 1999;319:1054–9.

[2] Hankins GD, Speer M. Defining the pathogenesis and pathophysiology of neonatal encephalopathy and cerebral palsy. Obstet Gynecol 2003;102:628–36.

[3] Eisenberg MS, Cummins RO, Ho MT. Code blue: cardiac arrest and resuscitation. Philadelphia: Saunders; 1987. p. 146.

[4] ACOG Committee on Obstetric Practice. ACOG Committee Opinion No. 348, November 2006: umbilical cord blood gas and acid-base analysis. Obstet Gynecol 2006;108:1319–22.

[5] Waugh J, Johnson A, Farkas A. Analysis of cord blood gas at delivery: questionnaire study of practice in the United Kingdom. BMJ 2001;323:727.

[6] Royal College of Obstetricians and Gynaecologists; Royal College of Midwives. Towards safer childbirth. Minimum standards for the organisation of labour wards. Report of a joint working party. London: RCOG Press; 1999. p. 22.

[7] Westgate J, Garibaldi JM, Greene KR. Umbilical cord blood gas analysis at delivery: a time for quality data. Br J Obstet Gynaecol 1994;101:1054–63.

[8] Nodwell A, Carmichael L, Ross M, et al. Placental compared with umbilical cord blood to assess fetal blood gas and acid-base status. Obstet Gynecol 2005;105:129–38.

[9] Perlman S, Goldman RD, Maatuk H, et al. Is the sampling site along the umbilical artery significant? Gynecol Obstet Invest 2002;54:172–5.

[10] Hilger JS, Holzman IR, Brown DR. Sequential changes in placental blood gases and pH during the hour following delivery. J Reprod Med 1981;26:305–7.

[11] Strickland DM, Gilstrap LC 3rd, Hauth JC, et al. Umbilical cord pH and PCO2: effect of interval from delivery to determination. Am J Obstet Gynecol 1984;148:191–4.

[12] Duerbeck NB, Chaffin DG, Seeds JW. A practical approach to umbilical artery pH and blood gas determinations. Obstet Gynecol 1992;79:959–62.

[13] Chauhan SP, Cowan BD, Meydrech EF, et al. Determination of fetal acidemia at birth from a remote umbilical arterial blood gas analysis. Am J Obstet Gynecol 1994;170:1705–9.

[14] Valenzuela P, Guijarro R. The effects of time on pH and gas values in the blood contained in the umbilical cord. Acta Obstet Gynecol Scand 2006;85:1307–9.

[15] Paerregaard A, Nickelsen CN, Brandi L, et al. The influence of sampling site and time upon umbilical cord blood acid-base status and PO2 in the newborn infant. J Perinat Med 1987; 15:559–63.

[16] Armstrong L, Stenson B. Effect of delayed sampling on umbilical cord arterial and venous lactate and blood gases in clamped and unclamped vessels. Arch Dis Child Fetal Neonatal Ed 2006;91:F342–5.

[17] Sato I, Saling E. Changes of pH-values during storage of fetal blood samples. J Perinat Med 1975;3:211–4.

[18] Manor M, Blickstein I, Hazan Y, et al. Postpartum determination of umbilical artery blood gases: effect of time and temperature. Clin Chem 1998;44:681–3.

[19] Sykes GS, Molloy PM. Effect of delays in collection or analysis on the results of umbilical cord blood measurements. Br J Obstet Gynaecol 1984;91:989–92.

[20] Pel M, Treffers PE. The reliability of the result of the umbilical cord pH. J Perinat Med 1983; 11:169–74.

ELSEVIER
SAUNDERS

CLINICS IN
PERINATOLOGY

Clin Perinatol 34 (2007) 461–471

Professional Misconduct and Ethics

Steven F. Seidman, MD, JD

*Heidell, Pittoni, Murphy & Bach, LLP, 99 Park Avenue, New York,
NY 10016, USA*

The Tenth Amendment of the United States Constitution empowers states to enact laws and regulations to protect its citizens' health, general welfare, and safety. Pursuant to this authority, states license and regulate physicians because of the potential harm that a licensed physician could cause its citizens as a result of incompetence, impairment, or moral turpitude [1]. State legislatures are empowered to specify what is considered forbidden physician conduct and are authorized to establish regulatory agencies to enforce physician compliance with laws established to safeguard quality statewide health care and assure appropriate behavior of physicians licensed to practice in that state.

Proscribed physician conduct, delineated by the legislature as professional misconduct, is extremely broad in scope and includes incompetence; reoccurring malpractice; dishonesty; deception; impairment by alcohol, drugs, physical disability, or mental disability; nonmedical criminal conduct, and so forth.

Conduct that raises ethical issues in the specialty of obstetrics and gynecology (and, specifically, in perinatology) does not necessarily amount to professional misconduct. Obstetricians often face conflicts involving patient (maternal) autonomy and fetal well-being. Although professional misconduct and ethics are separate entities, there are times when an obstetrician/gynecologist's conduct must be examined in the context of the ethical uncertainties in their specialty.

The Federation of State Medical Boards

The Federation of State Medical Boards was established in 1912 to regulate the practice of medicine. The Federation of State Medical Boards has grown to currently include 70 state medical boards in the United States and its

E-mail address: SFS7249@aol.com

0095-5108/07/$ - see front matter © 2007 Elsevier Inc. All rights reserved.
doi:10.1016/j.clp.2007.03.015

territories and 14 state boards of osteopathic medicine [2]. The Federation of State Medical Boards recognized early on that to improve the safety, integrity, and quality of health care nationally, uniform guidelines would have to be established. Ultimately, these guidelines were incorporated into what later became known as the "Essentials of a Modern Medical Practice Act," which was first published in 1956 [2].

The first and subsequent editions of the "Essentials of a Modern Medical Practice Act" authorized the formation of state medical boards whose function was to enforce legislation enacted to regulate medical practice. As a result, individual state medical boards became responsible for (1) licensing physicians practicing within the state; (2) reregistering physicians to evaluate whether they maintained continued competence and adhered to ethical standards of practice; (3) investigating complaints relating to quality of care issues and physician conduct; (4) disciplining physicians whose actions violated state laws; (5) conducting evaluations of physicians' practice patterns and professional behavior, when indicated; and (6) overseeing the rehabilitation of physicians found to be impaired [1]. These functions were undertaken by the individual state medical boards to ensure compliance with the medical board's rules and regulations, state law, and appropriate standards of care.

Enforcement of laws and regulations defining misconduct

State legislatures enact laws to define professional misconduct, but the responsibility for enforcing these laws belongs to the individual state medical boards. Individual boards are also authorized to establish their own regulations, the enforcement of which is under their control. These laws and regulations define a broad spectrum of professional medical misconduct that is generic in nature and does not apply specifically to any one specialty (with the exception of psychiatrists who are held to more stringent standards in the case of physical contact or emotional involvement with patients that is construed as even remotely sexual). Legislatures identify an extensive list of activities in which a physician might engage that constitute professional misconduct. New York State, for example, delineates 47 separate activities in its Education Law that rise to the level of professional misconduct [3]. Any licensed physician found guilty of such misconduct is subject to discipline, which is customarily imposed by the state medical board or a branch of the state's department of public health.

Penalties for professional misconduct

When it has been determined that a physician has engaged in professional misconduct, punishment is imposed commensurate with its seriousness, whether patient harm has taken place or if the misconduct has the potential to cause such harm. In the case of misconduct resulting in patient injury or involving significant moral turpitude, the medical board might determine that the appropriate penalty is license suspension or revocation [4]. In the case of less egregious misconduct, state boards have elected not to take action against the physician's license, instead mandating that the physician engage in additional education, training, monitoring, or a combination of these activities. The spectrum of penalties imposed by medical boards in the case of professional misconduct includes the following [4]:

1. Reprimand or censure—the physician is reprimanded for his or her conduct; this may become public record
2. Administrative fine—as per medical board mandate, the physician is required to pay a civil fine
3. Restitution—the physician is ordered to repay money that has been improperly earned to a patient or other entity (eg, insurance carrier)
4. Probation—the board monitors the physician's conduct, license, or both for a specified period to assure that misconduct does not reoccur
5. Limitation or restriction—limitations are placed on the physician's practice preventing the physician from engaging in specified procedures or engaging in medical practice without supervision
6. Suspension—the physician is prohibited from practicing medicine for a stated period
7. Summary suspension—the board makes the determination that the physician's continued practice of medicine constitutes a public health hazard and immediately suspends the physician from practicing
8. Voluntary license surrender—the physician "voluntarily" turns in his or her medical license to avoid board-imposed disciplinary action
9. Denial—the board determines that a physician's medical license will not be renewed
10. Revocation—the physician's license is terminated, and the physician can no longer practice

Relationship between state medical boards and the American College of Obstetricians and Gynecologists

Although state medical boards share information about disciplinary actions imposed on physicians, the relationship between state medical boards and the American College of Obstetricians and Gynecologists (ACOG) is different. State medical boards do not report licensure actions taken against ACOG members to ACOG itself. Similarly, when the ACOG learns that an ACOG member has engaged in activities that might rise to the level of professional misconduct, the ACOG is not required to report the member's misconduct to the respective state medical boards in which that physician is licensed.

The American College of Obstetricians and Gynecologists Grievance Committee

Nevertheless, the ACOG monitors actions taken against its members by individual state medical boards. The ACOG Grievance Committee pursues and reviews medical board actions taken as a result of professional conduct that violates ACOG's Code of Professional Ethics or is inconsistent with its bylaw requirements for admission [5]. In this regard, the ACOG Grievance Committee reviews all serious disciplinary actions imposed by medical boards, including but not limited to license revocation or suspension and all cases in which there has been a finding of sexual misconduct [5]. Not all licensure actions imposed by state medical boards result in expulsion from ACOG. If the board's findings are sustained, however, ACOG's bylaws authorize the following possible sanctions: warning, censure, suspension, or expulsion [5].

The ACOG Grievance Committee not only reviews and evaluates state medical board actions, it is also empowered by the bylaws to assess any complaints that a College Fellow might bring regarding the professional conduct of another Fellow of the College potentially in violation of ACOG's Code of Professional Ethics [6]. ACOG Grievance Committee hearing panels are composed of current or former members of the Committee and are responsible for evaluating such complaints. The committee determines whether the complaints should be sustained. In cases in which the complaint is found to be valid, the ACOG Grievance Committee recommends disciplinary action to the ACOG's executive board [6].

In addition, the ACOG Grievance Committee is empowered to make recommendations to the executive committee regarding the scope of its activities and to make recommendations targeted at the ACOG's grievance policy itself [6]. ACOG Grievance Committee members can also act as a hearing panel for ACOG applicants whose application for membership has been denied.

The American College of Obstetricians and Gynecologists code of professional ethics and statutory misconduct

The ACOG has published its own overview of ethical conduct that addresses numerous situations unique to practicing obstetrician-gynecologists titled *Ethics in Obstetrics and Gynecology* [7]. According to the ACOG, the purpose of this publication was to "help obstetrician-gynecologists understand and apply the concepts of biomedical ethics to problems in clinical practice, research, and the provision of health care in the community" [7]. Certain deviations from ethical conduct, as cited by ACOG, also amount to professional misconduct according to standards espoused by the Federation of State Medical Boards. These actions include physician conduct that negatively impacts patient safety, welfare, or the patient–physician relationship [8].

The Federation of State Medical Boards' Special Committee on Professional Conduct has recognized that professional organizations (eg, ACOG)—separate and apart from state medical boards—make modifications and amendments to their individual codes of ethics codes that are "beyond the control of the medical board[s]"[8]. For this reason, the Federation of State Medical Boards' Special Committee on Professional Conduct and Ethics has taken the position that state boards advocate compliance with the recognized codes of ethics promulgated by the American Medical Association and the American Osteopathic Association and not extend statutory authority to ethics codes established by individual practice specialties [8]. Therefore, unless an ethical violation identified by the ACOG or other professional medical organization also amounts to statutory professional misconduct (the enforcement of which lies within the state medical board's purview), that medical organization's disciplinary authority will extend only to its own members.

For ease of use, the 2004 edition of *Ethics in Obstetrics and Gynecology* has grouped related ethical obligations together [7]. Parts I, III, and IV are described briefly here. Part II touches on several ethical issues relevant to perinatology, and a more in-depth review of these issues follows. Part I, entitled "Ethical Foundations," includes a stepwise format for making ethical decisions in the practice of obstetrics and gynecology; addresses common issues faced in daily practice; and provides detailed information explaining the rationale for obtaining informed consent, offering practical assistance in how this may be accomplished [7]. Part III deals with professional responsibilities and examines the critical topic of sexual misconduct involving obstetricians-gynecologists and their patients. In Part IV, the ethical implications of obstetricians-gynecologists' societal responsibilities are reviewed. These responsibilities include relationships with industry (especially when there is a conflict between financial gain resulting from such relationships and the quality of patient care) and responsibilities inherent in providing expert testimony [7].

Part II of *Ethics in Obstetrics and Gynecology*, whose relevance to perinatology-related ethical issues has already been noted, is titled "Caring for Patients." Most issues raised in Part II do not subject the obstetrician-gynecologist to charges of professional misconduct but raise moral conundrums, nonetheless. This section begins by describing a process that provides obstetrician-gynecologists with guidance in making ethical decisions regarding surgical procedures specific to the specialty [7]. The procedures examined span the beginning to the end of life and include the unique maternal–fetal relationship [7]. Additional topics included in Part II review patient testing, patient choice in the maternal–fetal relationship, sex selection, and multifetal pregnancy reduction [7]. Also found here is the ACOG Committee Opinion examining maternal decision making, ethics, and the law [9].

Ethical principles in obstetrics and gynecology

According to the principles promulgated in *Ethics in Obstetrics and Gynecology* [7], there are five overriding ethical principles in obstetrics and gynecology:

1. respect for patient autonomy;
2. beneficence;
3. nonmaleficence;
4. justice; and
5. veracity.

Patient autonomy and informed consent (or refusal) are crucial to the question of whether there has been actual patient choice in choosing one treatment option over another. The obligation to inform the patient of additional treatment modalities and the potential risks and benefits of each rests exclusively with the clinical obstetrician-gynecologist. When (and not until) the physician is confident that the patient fully understands her treatment options, the patient's autonomous choice should customarily be respected. This does not mean that the obstetrician-gynecologist must necessarily agree with the choice made by the patient. When the patient's choice of treatment options conflicts with the other four ethical principles, "these other principles may take priority over supporting the patient's decision" [10].

The ethical principle of beneficence relates to the physician's responsibility to foster patient health and welfare. The ethical principle of nonmaleficence is the complimentary responsibility of physicians to not harm their patients. There is always the chance that a patient's autonomy will conflict with the physician's beneficence and nonmaleficence when the patient refuses a treatment option that, in the physician's opinion, would positively impact the patient's health and welfare. Even though patients almost always have the right to refuse treatment, they do not have the "parallel right to demand treatment that the physician believes is unwise or overly risky" [10].

From the medical perspective, the ethical principle of justice requires that a physician treat everyone fairly (not just patients) in performing professional responsibilities. The ethical principle of veracity refers to the physician's responsibility to tell the truth (eg, not misrepresent to a patient the physician's experience in performing a proposed surgical procedure or the success rate achieved when performing that procedure) [10].

The unique maternal–fetal relationship and the ethical issues posed when an obstetrician-gynecologist provides care to a parturient are examined in a recent ACOG Committee Opinion [9] and in the second part of *Ethics in Obstetrics and Gynecology* [7]. The maternal–fetal relationship is unlike any other faced by physicians due to the fetus' complete physiologic dependence on the mother and because both the fetus and mother are considered patients of the obstetrician. Furthermore, to therapeutically intervene on behalf of the fetus, the obstetrician has no choice but to accomplish this intervention through the parturient's body. The parturient, in turn, may sustain bodily harm resulting from such intervention even though the purpose was to benefit fetal outcome (not maternal well-being) [11]. In the case of virtually all pregnant women, fetal well-being is of utmost concern. Situations exist, however, in which maternal and fetal interests are opposed. First, there is the situation in which a mother refuses a diagnostic or therapeutic intervention whose sole purpose is to benefit fetal outcome. A second situation in which maternal and fetal interests diverge involves maternal behaviors that are harmful to the fetus.

Quality medical care has always focused on achieving greatest benefit while minimizing the risk of patient harm. This standard can become clouded in the case of a parturient and her fetus because the woman might value potential risks and benefits differently than the obstetrician who is acting on behalf of the fetus' well-being. When fetal welfare is imperiled, the mother is often asked to undergo diagnostic or therapeutic procedures not for her own benefit but to improve fetal outcome. Examples of this conundrum include a mother who undergoes a cesarean section for fetal distress or intrauterine fetal transfusion for isoimmunization [12]. Another situation in which maternal and fetal interests diverge occurs when the parturient engages in behaviors such as smoking or recreational drug use that negatively impact fetal welfare. In situations such as these, the woman is asked to modify her behavior to improve fetal outcome.

But what are the obstetrician's ethical obligations when the parturient refuses to undergo diagnostic or therapeutic procedures clinically indicated to improve fetal outcome or refuses to modify/cease engaging in behaviors recognized as harmful to the fetus? Is it ethical for the obstetrician to allow a pregnant patient to refuse treatment and thereby imperil fetal outcome? On the other hand, should the obstetrician force the parturient to undergo a therapeutic procedure involuntarily in the hope of positively impacting fetal well-being? These ethical issues are complicated by two concerns that the obstetrician must always face:

1. Should the parturient and the fetus be treated as individual patients?
2. Should the interests of the parturient and the fetus be treated as divergent or shared?

Recent legal actions and policies have attempted to protect the fetus as an entity separate from the mother. These legal actions and policies have challenged the parturient's right to decide whether she will undergo therapeutic interventions or modify certain behaviors to improve fetal outcome. Some recent legal decisions that are focused on improving fetal well-being have even imposed criminal sanctions on maternal behaviors such as cigarette smoking and recreational drug use, which are thought to contribute to poor perinatal outcomes [9].

On occasion, physicians and hospital representatives, hoping to positively impact fetal outcome, have instituted legal actions in an attempt to have the courts order parturients to undergo therapeutic procedures that the parturient previously refused [9]. Ethical issues arose, however, when the court's directive, issued for the presumed benefit of the fetus, was contrary to the parturient's wishes [9].

Several lower courts throughout the country have had to rule on whether to compel a parturient to undergo a cesarean section, typically when the well-being of the fetus was at risk. In most of these cases, the court did order the parturient to undergo cesarean section [13]. Requests for court orders are often made at a critical point in the pregnancy, and the lower court must necessarily make a ruling soon after the request is first heard. Given the exigent, rushed circumstances surrounding the court's decision, the possibility of judicial error is substantial. These decisions are rarely appealed after the cesarean section has been completed because of disinterest or because the issue is now moot. As a result of the rushed circumstances that the court must face, there is often little time to examine legal precedents in formulating a decision. There are, however, two appellate decisions that examine the issues involved when a court is requested to order a parturient to involuntarily undergo a therapeutic intervention to positively impact fetal outcome [14].

One of these appellate decisions comes from the US Court of Appeals, District of Columbia Circuit (*In re A.C.*, A2d 1235 [D.C. Cir. 1990]). In this matter, the Court of Appeals overturned a lower court's decision giving a hospital permission to perform a cesarean section on a terminally ill parturient who was comatose. The parturient was expected to die soon, and the cesarean section was recommended only to salvage the fetus, not for any maternal benefit. In fact, physicians believed that the surgery itself would probably hasten the parturient's death. On appeal, the court based its analysis on the "tenet common to all medical treatment cases: that any person has the right to make an informed choice, if competent to do so, to accept or forego medical treatment" [15]. The Court of Appeals took the position that "one human being is under no legal compulsion to give aid or to take action to save another human being.... For our law to compel defendant [ie, the parturient] to submit to an intrusion of [her] body would change every concept and principle upon which our society is founded.... To do so would defeat the sanctity of the individual" [16]. The Court of Appeals concluded that if a competent patient has made an informed decision regarding the treatment course she wishes to pursue, then "that decision will control in virtually all cases" [17].

The parturient in *In re A.C.*, however, was not competent to make an informed decision whether to undergo cesarean section. Here, the Court of Appeals held that, in the case of a parturient who was incapable of giving informed consent to the proposed cesarean section, the lower court's duty was to act as the incompetent's surrogate and "determine as best it can what choice that individual, if competent, would make with respect to medical procedures" [18]. This analysis, known as the substituted judgment procedure, makes it the court's duty to act as a decision maker and "substitute itself as nearly as may be for the incompetent, and...act upon the same motives and considerations as would have moved her" [19].

The Georgia Supreme Court issued the other appellate decision on whether a parturient could be ordered to undergo a cesarean section involuntarily. The case, *Jefferson v Griffin Spalding County Hospital Authority*, involved a pregnant woman who had refused to undergo cesarean section for religious reasons [20]. The trial court held that the pregnant woman should undergo cesarean section because the fetus was viable and Georgia law made it illegal to abort a viable fetus. The trial court's authorization of the cesarean section, however, required the parturient to admit herself voluntarily to one of the County Hospitals. The Georgia Department of Human Resources found the hospital admission requirement unacceptable and requested the juvenile court to grant the Department of Human Resources temporary custody of the fetus and order the parturient to undergo cesarean section [21]. The juvenile court and Georgia Supreme Court hearings were consolidated and, on appeal, the appellate court ruled that, as a viable being, the fetus was entitled to protection under the state's child neglect statute. Holding that the state had "an interest in protecting the lives of unborn viable children," the appellate court explained that it had "weighed the right of the mother to practice her religion and to refuse surgery on herself, against her unborn child's right to live" and "found in favor of her child's right to live" [20].

The uncooperative parturient—ethical considerations

ACOG has identified three separate choices an obstetrician has when a competent parturient refuses to abide by medical recommendations despite reasonable attempts to educate and persuade the patient. The obstetrician can choose to respect the patient's autonomy and allow her to not comply with treatment recommendations despite potentially adverse effects on the fetus. The obstetrician's second possible course of action is to recommend to the parturient that she seek obstetric care from another provider before an emergent situation arises causing an irresolvable conflict between the patient and physician. This second option should be the choice of an obstetrician who is unwilling to permit the parturient to follow a course of action that is contrary to medical recommendations and that could negatively impact fetal outcome. The third and most infrequent option chosen by the obstetrician who is dealing with an uncooperative parturient is to request court intervention. Which option is ultimately chosen depends on "the urgency of the clinical circumstances, the potential consequences for both the pregnant woman and the fetus, and the reliability of predictions of such consequences" [11].

When dealing with noncompliant parturients, the ACOG has recommended that obstetricians consider three ethical principles when choosing among the options mentioned in the preceding paragraph. The first such principle involves the obstetrician's respect for the parturient's autonomy, which in essence, obligates the physician to respect the patient's decision whether she complies or rejects the physician's therapeutic recommendations. The second of these principles invokes the obstetrician's beneficence, which requires the physician to support measures improving the health and welfare of the parturient and the fetus. This second principle also obligates the parturient to promote fetal well-being. The third ethical principle the obstetrician must consider is that of justice, the duty to treat similarly situated people (parturient and nonparturient alike) in the same manner. Following this final principle, the obstetrician is reminded that all individuals have the right to refuse invasive therapeutic interventions, and this holds equally true for a parturient, who should not be compelled to undergo therapeutic interventions involuntarily to benefit fetal outcome [11].

ACOG's Committee on Ethics has taken the position that an obstetrician rarely is justified in obtaining a court-ordered directive compelling a parturient to involuntarily undergo therapeutic intervention for fetal benefit. The Committee on Ethics' position is that the following criteria must be met before an obstetrician should even begin considering court intervention to force a parturient to accept therapeutic intervention involuntarily [11]:

1. continuing to comply with the parturient's refusal of therapeutic intervention poses a risk of likely harm to the fetus;
2. the contemplated treatment that the parturient is refusing will, in all likelihood, reduce potential harm to the fetus;
3. tess-intrusive therapeutic options are not available; and
4. the recommended treatment poses insignificant risk to the parturient and may even benefit her.

Even in the event that these criteria are met, ACOG's Committee on Ethics believes that obstetricians must use restraint before seeking a court order to override the parturient's refusal to comply with medical recommendations. Forcing a pregnant woman to involuntarily undergo medical or surgical treatment in the hope of improving fetal outcome and thereby infringing on her autonomy cannot avoid creating animosity on the mother's part. At the very least, the parturient becomes distrustful of the health care system and the patient–physician relationship likely suffers irreparable harm. More uncertain are the psychologic effects on the parturient forced to undergo treatment against her wishes and how the woman's future use of the health care system will ultimately be impacted [11].

References

[1] Federation of State Medical Boards of the United States, Inc. Trends in physician regulation. Dallas: Federation of State Medical Boards of the United States; 2006, p. 14.

[2] Federation of State Medical Boards of the United States, Inc. Essentials of a modern medical practice act. 11th edition. Dallas: Federation of State Medical Boards of the United States; 2006. p. 1.

[3] New York State Education Law §6530.

[4] Federation of State Medical Boards of the United States, Inc. Protecting the public: how state medical boards regulate and discipline physicians. p. 1, 2. Available at: http://www.fsmb.org/smb_protecting_public.html. Accessed December 28, 2006.

[5] The American College of Obstetricians and Gynecologists. Discipline by state medical boards creates domino effect. May/June 2005. p. 14. Available at: http://www.acog.org/departments/dept_notice.cfm?recno=36&bulletin=3856. Accessed December 31, 2006.

[6] The American College of Obstetricians and Gynecologists. Grievance committee description. Available at: http://acog.org/departments/dept_notice.cfm?recno=46&bulletin=3870. Accessed January 10, 2007.

[7] The American College of Obstetrics and Gynecology. Ethics in obstetrics and gynecology. 2nd edition; Washington, DC; 2004. Available at: http://www.acog.org/from_home/publications/ethics/ethicsVII.cfm. Accessed January 31, 2007.

[8] Federation of State Medical Boards of the United States, Inc. Report of the special committee on professional conduct and ethics. Dallas: Federation of State Medical Boards of the United States; 2000. p. 2–4.

[9] The American College of Obstetrics and Gynecology. Maternal decision making, ethics, and the law. ACOG Committee Opinion No. 321. Obstet Gynecol 2005;106:1127–37.

[10] The American College of Obstetrics and Gynecology. Ethics in obstetrics and gynecology: surgery and patient choice. 2nd edition. Washington, DC: American College of Obstetrics and Gynecology; 2004. p. 21–2.

[11] The American College of Obstetrics and Gynecology. Ethics in obstetrics and gynecology: patient choice in the maternal-fetal relationship. 2nd edition. Washington, DC: American College of Obstetrics and Gynecology; 2004. p. 34.

[12] The American College of Obstetrics and Gynecology. Ethics in obstetrics and gynecology. 2nd edition. Washington, DC: American College of Obstetrics and Gynecology; 2004. p. 34–36.

[13] In re A.C., 533 A2d 611, 617 (DC 1987). [Upheld the trial court order compelling parturient to undergo cesarean section]; In re Madyun Fetus, 114 Daily Wash L Rep 2233 (DC Super Ct July 26, 1986). [Over mother's objection, court ordered the parturient to undergo a cesarean section to avoid fetal infection with resultant brain injury that might result after vaginal delivery. Court reasoned that it could order the cesarean section and override the competent mother's objection because the state had a compelling interest in preserving the fetus' life.]

[14] Eric M. Levine. Comments: the constitutionality of court ordered cesarean surgery: a threshold question, 4 Alb. L.J. Sci. & Tech 229:240.

[15] In re: A.C., 573 A2d 1235, 1243 (DC Cir 1990).

[16] In re: A.C., 573 A2d 1243-4 (DC Cir 1990).

[17] In re: A.C., 573 A2d 1249 (DC Cir 1990).

[18] In re: A.C., 573 A2d 1249 (DC Cir 1990) (quoting from In Re Boyd, 403 A2d 744, 750 [DC 1979]).

[19] In re: A.C., 573 A2d 1249 (DC Cir 1990) (quoting from City Bank Farmers Trust Co. v McGowan, 323 US 594, 599 [1945]).

[20] Jefferson v Grifin Spading County Hospital Authority, 247 Ga 86 (Ga 1981).

[21] Eric M. Levine. Comments: the constitutionality of court ordered cesarean surgery: a threshold question, 4 Alb. L.J. Sci. & Tech 229:246.

ELSEVIER
SAUNDERS

CLINICS IN
PERINATOLOGY

Clin Perinatol 34 (2007) 473–488

Expert Witness Testimony

Erol Amon, MD, JD

*Maternal-Fetal Medicine, Department of Obstetrics, Gynecology, and Women's Health,
Saint Louis University, 6420 Clayton Road, St. Louis, MO 63132, USA*

How can the jury judge between two statements each founded upon an experience confessedly foreign in kind to their own? It is just because they are incompetent for such a task that the expert is necessary at all.
—Judge Learned Hand

Medicine and law are two of mankind's greatest civilized undertakings. In many ways, they are similar. Analogous to the physician–patient relationship is the attorney–client relationship: physicians and attorneys share the duty of confidentiality and the duty to place patients' or clients' interests before their own self-interest. In most instances, the patient or client is in an extremely vulnerable position in need of professional assistance. This asymmetric relationship and profound levels of duty call for a very high degree of professionalism, which is expected from members of both professions.

In other ways, these two types of relationships are markedly different. Medicine employs an open, cooperative, yet tightly constrained scientific methodology interested in discovering the truth. In contrast, the American legal system uses a relatively hidden, more creative, adversarial approach in which the courts and jurors unearth the truth to the best of their abilities. The attorney's goal is to use the adversarial system to win his or her case rather than to search for truth. Although scientific studies generally advance a physician's goal to care for his or her patient, it may detract from the attorney's theory on a malpractice case. The attorney must counter this science because in all circumstances, attorneys have the ethical duty to advocate zealously for their client. Where scientific unknowns remain as unanswered questions without conclusions in medicine, legal disputes must always be conclusively decided on and finality reached regardless of the quality and quantity of evidence presented. Physicians are trained in the traditional sciences and its methodologies, whereas attorneys are generally schooled in methods of advocacy, debate, and political sciences [1].

E-mail address: amone@slucare1.sluh.edu

doi:10.1016/j.clp.2007.03.016   *perinatology.theclinics.com*

One of the most important interfaces between medicine and law occurs in the courtroom [2]. Most physicians are called on during their career to provide legal testimony in one context or another. They could be a party to a lawsuit as a plaintiff or a defendant. They could be a fact witness providing first-hand knowledge about a patient's condition, treatment, and records. In this capacity, personal testimony relates to what he or she did or did not observe, hear, or do in the course of events at legal issue. Physicians may also be called on to provide expert testimony and opine regarding past events relating to a malpractice lawsuit for which they often have no first-hand knowledge of the patient's condition or care. They could also be called on to predict future medical outcomes, including life expectancy, and in a psychiatric context, even whether a patient is dangerous enough (homicidal or suicidal) to be involuntarily committed.

From a layperson's perspective, a physician is not only one of societies most respected members but also extremely knowledgeable about the complexities and intricacies of the human body and the practice of medicine. On both these accounts, when medical issues are litigated, physicians have potential to make excellent witnesses. Nonetheless, the practical ability to communicate clearly to a layperson is essential.

When called on to testify, most physicians bring a high degree of professionalism to the legal process and play a very important role in the administration of justice [3]. Unequivocally, a patient injured by genuine medical malpractice needs to be compensated and receive every penny due them. When true malpractice has occurred, the individual (patient) and society (all of us) benefit by professional testimony that assists a court in reaching that conclusion [4].

The funding for the medical liability system in large part relies on professional liability insurance premiums. Premiums for professional liability insurance increase according to the amounts of money needed to administer the insurance programs, to pay for defense attorneys and defense experts, and to pay any indemnity awarded to the plaintiff by a court or that is contractually settled on by both parties. Liability premiums escalate in response to the number of meritless suits resulting in zero payment to the plaintiff and the suits in which indemnity (which is increasing) is paid. As premiums rise, some physicians cannot afford to stay in the market, and access to lifesaving health care is diminished. Thus, the quantity and quality of medical malpractice lawsuits translates, to a reasonable extent, to the availability of medical care [4].

Integral to any medical malpractice lawsuit is the expert witness. This article reviews the law of professional negligence, the proper role, qualifications, and ethical requirements of expert witnesses, and the regulation of unprofessional testimony. Expert witness reform is also briefly discussed.

The law of professional negligence

The plaintiff has the burden of proof. In criminal cases, the burden to overcome is to provide evidence that is "beyond a reasonable doubt," which could be thought of as a 95% likelihood. Here, a defendant's life or liberty is at stake. In end-of-life cases in which a plaintiff requests removal of life support, courts often follow Supreme Court precedent in *Cruzan v Director, Missouri Department of Health* and apply a lower burden known as "clear and convincing evidence" [5], which could be thought of as a 67% likelihood. In professional negligence cases in which the remedy for injury due to an act of negligence is money, however, the court applies a mere "preponderance of the evidence" standard [6], which often equates to only a 51% likelihood or, as commonly construed, as "more likely than not."

The four elements that must be proved in professional negligence lawsuits are duty, breach, causation, and injury. Each element must be proved by the preponderance of evidence standard [2].

The first of these elements, a legal duty, is created by the physician–patient relationship. The duty arising out of this relationship is to provide standard medical care that would be exercised by other reasonable similarly situated physicians under similar circumstances [6]. These standards of care refer to appropriate conduct (ie, behavior—actions or inactions of the defendant). The standards of care do not refer to a mindset (ie, character) to harm or help the plaintiff.

It is noteworthy to contrast a legal duty from an ethical duty. A legal duty is what must or must not be done that a court of law may (or will) enforce. An ethical duty is what someone should or should not do, and a court may not (or will not) find it enforceable. Consider a physician who happens to be shopping at a mall and the person standing in front of him collapses and stops breathing. The physician ethically should assist that person; however, in the absence of a pre-existing physician–patient relationship, he has no legal duty or legal requirement to help and cannot be hailed into a court for failing to provide medical care. When this physician takes action to help, however, he must do it non-negligently. To encourage these selfless acts, almost all states have enacted "Good Samaritan statutes" to protect these good people from lawsuits [7].

The second element to be proved by the plaintiff is the defendant's breach of the standard of care (the legal duty). Here, the physician's conduct is at issue. The negligent (ie, breached) conduct is an omission of an owed duty or commission of a negligent act. To prove this element, expert witness testimony is generally required to provide admissible evidence for the benefit of the court by answering two questions: (1) What is or should have been the standard of medical care? and (2) Was the duty to provide that standard breached by the defendant physician? [2].

The legal principle of *res ipsa loquitor* is an exception to the plaintiff's requirement for expert witness testimony. This legal doctrine addresses the adverse outcome that could only have come about by the defendant's negligence. It is a rule of circumstantial proof [6]. A prime example is the unintentional leaving of a sponge in a patient's abdomen after a surgical procedure. Here, the layperson may use common sense and reason that this was clearly negligence. In this clear-cut situation, the judge would likely agree that expert physician testimony unnecessary.

The third element of proof is legal causation. There must be a reasonably close and causal connection between the breach of the standard and the alleged injury. The legal question asked and answered by the expert is "but for the defendant's breach, would the plaintiff have suffered the injury?" [6]. In other words, the breach must be a necessary condition that leads to the injury. Furthermore, the attorney is often required to ask the expert witness whether the alleged breach resulted in the alleged injury "within a reasonable degree of medical certainty" [2].

This notion of legal cause is generally different from medical causation. In medicine, causation is complex and depends on multiple factors. To establish scientific proof using evidenced-based medicine, physicians often rely on controlled clinical trials with mathematic probabilities that strive to explain the observed results by isolating the study ie, experimental variable and by minimizing the occurrence of happenstance or chance. Causation is further strengthened when these results are independently reproducible.

In law, however, the focus is not scientific truth. The heart of the matter is the attribution of responsibility [8]. Therefore, by necessity, the law commences a retrospective investigation of the particular conduct of particular persons. Evidence law states that evidence is relevant if it has "any tendency to make the existence of any fact that is of consequence to the determination of the action more probable or less probable than it would be without the evidence" [9]. This evidence must be pertinent to the case and help the jury make a final decision. Here, the 51% standard is clearly being invoked to persuade the jury of causation.

The final element that requires legal proof is the development of an injury. The purpose of awarding monetary damages is to make the victim "whole, " legally speaking. If there is no injury, then there is no recovery on which damages can be based. Compensatory damages are usually of two types: economic (measurable) and noneconomic (nonmeasurable). Economic damages include case-related past, present, and future medical expenses and related loss of past, present, and future wages. An economic expert in life planning will testify as to the amount of economic damages. Noneconomic damages include those related to "pain and suffering," loss of consortium, and mental anguish. It is unfortunate that these damages cannot be accurately quantified and are thus subject to a sizable degree of variation among juries. Many state legislatures, through tort law reforms, have enacted a hard cap on noneconomic damages to protect against runaway jury awards, to improve the predictability of judgment amounts, and to stabilize insurance premiums and maintain access to medical care [4].

Ultimately, all four elements must be linked together for the plaintiff to prevail, with each element being proved by a preponderance of the evidence [2]. When a physician defendant has no legal duty to the patient, the suit will fail to go forward. When the defendant can show that the standard of care was met despite an adverse outcome (maloccurrence), the defendant should prevail. If the defendant breached a standard of medical care owed to the plaintiff, but the breach did not cause or was unrelated to the injury, then the plaintiff should not be able to recover any damages.

Legal duty is hardly ever litigated because in most cases, there is usually a well-defined physician–patient relationship. On the other hand, evidence of the last three elements is often controversial, often litigated, and most often introduced into court through the testimony of experts.

Multiple experts may be used to prove each element independently. In contrast to fact witnesses, experts are the only witnesses permitted to reflect, opine, and pontificate in court. Initially, a standard-of-care expert introduces testimony and educates the jury on what the appropriate medical practice is or should be and whether the defendant's conduct falls within the standard of care. Causation experts may be used to establish whether the alleged breach legally caused the alleged injury "within a reasonable degree of medical certainty." Economic experts may argue over the degree of damages, life expectancy, and projected future costs. Most attorneys recognize that proving liability is one thing, but getting all the damages claimed is another.

An expert is defined as a person who, by reason of education or special training, possesses knowledge of a particular subject area at greater depth than the judge or lay jury. The judge will often decide on the admissibility of this evidence (the expert's testimony) by assessing the proffered expert's qualifications and opposing counsel's objections. When the expert is allowed to testify in the courtroom, the jury will weigh the testimony about his or her interpretation (opinions) of the facts of the case.

The adversarial battleground

The American legal system is known as the adversarial system. Originating in English law, the adversarial system relies on opposing parties and their attorneys to investigate, prosecute, and defend the parties by collecting, organizing, and presenting the evidence [10]. Opposing attorneys examine and cross-examine the witnesses and, by using the rules of evidence, attempt to convince an impartial and relatively passive court of the correctness of their clients' position. The other dominant legal system, which seeks a just remedy, is the inquisitorial system in which the judiciary is proactive and does the questioning of witnesses. For the most part, this approach is not used in the United States civil justice system.

The adversarial system of litigation is the cornerstone of the American justice system. Ideally, if two equally matched (by intelligence, experience, and resources) attorneys zealously and competently represent their clients within the bounds of ethical and legal rules and if there are perfectly neutral judges and juries, then the correct result should be reached.

The reasoned basis for the adversarial system is that true facts will emerge under a vigorous attempt of each party to advance its own favorable evidence (interpretation of historical facts) while attempting to limit admissibility or limit the credibility of its opponent's evidence. The trier of fact (judge or jury) assesses the evidence and unearths the "real truth." Ultimately, a conclusion must be reached and one side loses.

In this system, however, there is no obligation to present all the facts—only those favorable to a particular side. The attorneys are not under oath. The judge often does not take an active role and simply remains a neutral referee ruling on admissibility of evidence and other legal issues as they arise. Each side is presumed to look after their own interests and to define the scope of relevant evidence. The court is not interested in reviewing evidence that the parties do not present. Jurors are also passive participants who are usually unable to ask clarifying questions [11].

Expert witnesses for both sides present their opinions regarding the evidence previously produced. Moreover, the expert offers his or her opinion as evidence. Testimonial and other evidence is tightly controlled and shaped to various degrees by the opposing attorneys. As a result (and not infrequently), it is an incomplete view of the truth.

There are important stages that evidence will pass through: the witness must be located and induced to testify, the witness must be prepared for testifying, the testimony must be presented, and the testimony must be evaluated [11].

Gross [11] described the inevitable process as follows. Opposing attorneys select experts who will advance or develop their theory of the case. The expert need not have any previous contact or previous knowledge of the case; however, he or she needs to be other than minimally qualified by minimal legal requirements. Experts are often selected from a large pool, not based on an impartial assessment or expert stature but based on what they will say and how they will say it. Next, the expert witness is highly remunerated by the hiring counsel. These witnesses become too readily available, and many advertise their services. Experts whose incomes depend heavily on testimony tend to please; otherwise, they would not be rehired or recommended for future cases.

Worst of all, this system of expert witness selection breeds contempt from lawyers, judges, and other physicians. Concurrently, it breeds contempt for the adversarial system of law and its lawyers. The impartial or unfavorable expert view may even be deselected in preference of another. Being highly remunerated and eager for recommendations or repeat engagements by the hiring attorney may explain why the expert witness may shift from objectivity and become an advocate for his or her side [11].

In obstetric cases with neurologic birth injuries, a relatively small group of physician experts testifies in a large portion of these cases. Furthermore, theses witnesses tend to establish themselves as plaintiff or defendant witnesses fairly consistently [12].

The lawyer in the adversarial system is a purveyor of evidence. The lawyer's responsibility is to present evidence—only the evidence that favors his side—and to present it skillfully. A lawyer who intends to present an expert for testimony prepares the witness to his or her benefit. As a result, the expert may spend significant time preparing to testify, especially if the situation is complex [11].

As the preparation takes place, the expert has a motive to construct defenses against the opposing lawyers because the work is done in anticipation of battle, under threat of attack. The expert is subject to camaraderie when working on a difficult project. The expert may become dependent on the lawyer for preparation to make his or her testimony successful and to seek protection against a formidable enemy. Hours of this type of preparation, perhaps more than payment, may push the expert to identify with his litigation team. In deposition preparation, experts for both sides may be instructed to not volunteer information and to view litigation as a fight in which he or she must take sides [11].

Proffered evidence is often probed for uncertainty, unreliability, bias, inconsistency, ability to mislead, and lack of relevance. On cross-examination, an attorney may ask leading (misleading) questions in such a manner and form as to be testifying while asking a series of very narrow questions, advancing his or her client's viewpoint. This practice can often lead to simplified, abbreviated, and distorted answers by the expert [11].

Furthermore, on cross-examination, physician witnesses can be aggressively challenged with personal attacks on their fund of knowledge, their objectiveness, their competency, their credentials, their character, and endurance. Aggressive cross-examination should be expected from opposing counsel because the attorney hopes that the expert witness will be rattled and lose his or her cool. Such cross-examination is all done in an attempt to diminish the impact of the opposing expert's testimony. This confrontation should be met with a high degree of professionalism and poise, but could be met with varying degrees of anger and argumentation depending on the witnesses' personal sense of resentment.

Clearly, selection, financial pressure, and biasing by partisan preparation by the hiring attorney, together with being placed in a defensive posture by anticipating aggressive attacks from the opposing attorney, conspire against the impartial and objective expert testimony. Hence, we have all the ingredients for a "battle of the experts" on an adversarial battleground.

The problem of conflicting experts and the battle of the experts was summed up in a 1901 article by Judge Learned Hand in a paradox: [13] "how can we expect jurors to decide between experts when the jurors' ignorance is the premise for allowing the expert to testify in the first place?" Furthermore, "One thing is for certain, they will do no better with the so-called testimony of experts than without, except where it is unanimous."

To truly assist in the administration of justice, the expert should be taught the partisan imperfections inherent in the adversarial system

[11–14]. Most important, an expert must bring to bear the positive forces of integrity, responsibility, professionalism, and ethics. The truth should be told candidly to the hiring attorney. Ideally, the expert should approach every question with independence and objectivity. Professional expert testimony should rise above selection and financial pressures. Partisan preparation (and resulting identification with a party) is a more subtle form of hiring an expert advocate and is more difficult to counter. Nonetheless, meeting certain qualifications and following certain ethical guidelines should assist the quest for objectivity.

Qualifications and ethical principles for the expert

In an attempt to promote the integrity of the individual expert witness and his or her professional organization, the following qualifications are recommended.

In general, an expert can be qualified by knowledge, skill, experience, training, or education; however, specific qualifications may vary from state to state and among professional organizations. According to the American College of Obstetricians and Gynecologists [15], the following are the qualifications of a physician expert witness:

1. The physician expert witness must have a current, valid, and unrestricted license to practice medicine in the state in which he or she practices.
2. The physician expert witness should be currently certified by a board recognized by the American Board of Medical Specialties and have experience or demonstrated competence in the subject of the case.
3. The specialty, training, and experience of the physician expert witness should be appropriate to the subject matter in the case.
4. The physician expert witness should be familiar with the standard of care provided at the time of the alleged occurrence. In addition, the physician expert witness should have been actively involved in the clinical practice of the specialty or the subject matter of the case within 5 years from the time the expert was retained to provide an expert opinion in the matter.
5. The physician expert witness should be able to demonstrate evidence of continuing medical education relevant to the specialty or the subject matter of the case.
6. The physician expert should be prepared to document the percentage of time that is involved in serving as an expert witness. In addition, the physician expert should be willing to disclose the amount of fees or compensation obtained for such activities and the total number of times the physician expert has testified for the plaintiff or defendant.

Furthermore, it is the duty of the expert witness to testify ethically on behalf of the plaintiffs and the defendants [16]. The expert should distinguish maloccurrence from malpractice. Maloccurrence is an adverse outcome unrelated to the quality of care provided, whereas malpractice is substandard care that causes harm. It is unethical for a physician expert to accept compensation that is contingent on the outcome of litigation [3]. The following are additional ethical principles for expert testimony:

1. The physician's review of medical facts must be thorough, fair, and impartial and must not exclude any relevant information. It must not be biased to create a view favoring the plaintiff, the government, or the defendant. The goal of a physician testifying in any judicial proceeding should be to provide testimony that is complete, objective, and helpful to a just resolution of the proceeding.
2. The physician's testimony must reflect an evaluation of performance in light of generally accepted standards, neither condemning performance that falls within generally accepted practice standards nor endorsing or condoning performance that falls below these standards. Medical decisions often must be made in the absence of diagnostic and prognostic certainty.
3. The physician must make every effort to assess the relationship of the alleged substandard practice to the outcome, because deviation from a practice standard is not always substandard care or causally related to a bad outcome.

Finally, the physician must be prepared to have testimony given in any judicial proceeding subjected to peer review by an institution or professional organization to which he or she belongs [16].

Regulating unprofessional testimony

Despite the preceding descriptions for qualified and ethical testimony, not surprisingly, unprofessional testimonial conduct still occurs. Some expert witnesses may misstate or misrepresent their credentials or knowingly misrepresent the standard of care. They may not be current in the area of claimed expertise or may not acknowledge other legitimate approaches to the liability issue in question. Our system of law should proactively deal with false or faulty testimony, but how? There are essentially three general approaches to regulating unprofessional testimony: the use of the courts, state licensing boards, and professional organizations [17].

Courts

The major formal guarantee of candor in the courtroom is the oath, "a solemn appeal to the Deity, made binding on the conscience by a penalty for perjury" [11]. Witnesses are required to swear to make lying a crime. Of note, lawyers advocating for their side in the courtroom are not under oath and may adeptly mislead the opposing witness, misspeak, or misread evidence to serve their clients' purpose.

Lying is not the only way that a witness can deceive; it is probably not even the major way. Witnesses frequently make mistakes, and they may color their testimony to a considerable extent without actually committing perjury. Nor does the oath impose a duty to provide complete evidence. A witness may swear to tell "the whole truth," but all she is actually obligated (and perhaps allowed by the attorneys) to do is give an honest answer to each question she is asked [11].

A criminal conviction for perjury is not easy. Perjury requires a specific, knowing intent to deceive, which makes it a notoriously difficult crime to prove, and even when it is suspected, it often has a low claim on prosecutorial resources. On rare occasions, there is a willingness to bring a criminal perjury action, especially if the offended party is the government [18]. Nonetheless, a systemic lack of perjury allegations reflects a diffuse legal approach that intimates it is better to let some liars get away with it than to discourage honest testimony by making the threat of prosecution for perjury too menacing [11].

Furthermore, most courts invoke the concept of witness immunity to encourage open and honest testimony without fear of reprisals or subsequent lawsuits based on the testimony provided. Otherwise, it would be inevitable that those who lose would pin the blame on witnesses and bring suit against them [19].

The judicial system seems to believe that its own internal machinery is adequate to ferret out abuse. It consists of taking an oath, using aggressive cross-examination, and observing witness manner, demeanor, appearance, responsiveness, and other indicia of credibility. It is thought that these factors (rather than substantive content) enables the trier of fact to determine the truthfulness of contrary expert testimony and, it is hoped, distinguish professional from unprofessional testimonial conduct. Cross-examination is aimed at impeaching witness credibility or discrediting the facts and conclusions presented by the expert.

Indeed, the US Supreme Court in Daubert [20] stated that vigorous cross-examination, presentation of contrary evidence, and careful jury instruction on burden of proof are the appropriate means of attacking shaky but admissible evidence (testimony).

The Court of Appeals Seventh Circuit indicates that public policy requires that witnesses who are a necessary part of the judicial system be privileged against any restraint except the penalty imposed by perjury. The Court of Appeals considers that the functioning of a tribunal would be seriously handicapped if witnesses, expert or otherwise, fear liability from statements made by them within the scope of litigation [21].

Clearly, courts prefer to sift the truth from masses of contrary evidence using its litigation machinery than to punish unprofessional testimony. Moreover, it seems that courts cannot easily keep out unprofessional testimony at the outset of a case. The chief judge of the US Court of Appeals Seventh Circuit, Richard Posner, referring to unprofessional expert testimony [22], wrote the following:

> It is no answer that judges can be trusted to keep out such testimony. Judges are not experts in any field except law. Much escapes us, especially in a highly technical field, such as neurosurgery. When a member of a prestigious professional association makes representations not on their face absurd, such as that a majority of neurosurgeons believe that a particular type of mishap is invariably the result of surgical negligence, the judge may have no basis for questioning the belief, even if the defendant's expert witness testifies to the contrary.

The credibility of experts in court is often decided on by superficial proxies of witness observation rather than the merits of the testimony itself. Manner, background, appearance, and presentation techniques seem to matter, with the focus on the messenger rather than the message. For the most part, and for reasons that are unclear, courts seem to promote the ideals and beneficiaries of the adversarial system, and courts rarely punish the unprofessional expert witness.

State licensing boards

The second major approach to the regulation of unprofessional testimony is through the state medical licensing board, composed primarily of governmentally appointed physicians of various disciplines. The boards are charged with protecting the public from incompetent, unprofessional, and unethical physician practices. Accordingly, the boards are required to (1) set up the entry criteria for a state licensure to practice medicine, (2) define the standards of professional medical conduct, and (3) enforce disciplinary measures when these standards are violated [23].

Statutes in each state enable these disciplinary acts. Typical grounds for discipline include obtaining a license to practice medicine by fraud, deceit, or misrepresentation; practicing medicine fraudulently or incompetently; practicing medicine while under the influence of alcohol or drugs or a physical or mental disability; habitual addiction to alcohol or narcotics; conviction of a crime; engaging in dishonorable, immoral, or unprofessional conduct; or violating the rules of the state medical board.

As such, unprofessional or false expert witness testimony may be regulated by these governmental medical licensing agencies. These boards can use their lawful power to sanction unprofessional and unethical medical practice in a progressive manner, from private reprimands to license revocation.

Currently, states differ in their interpretation of whether expert witness testimony constitutes the practice of medicine and is therefore within the ambit of regulation by state licensing boards. A 1997 survey found that most medical boards do not believe that giving expert witness testimony constitutes the practice of medicine [24]. Of the respondents, 41% expressed uncertainty as to whether a medical expert witness is "practicing medicine," and 72% had never disciplined a physician for fraudulent courtroom testimony [24].

Despite this decade-old survey, there is a growing trend among state medical boards indicating that by classifying the improper testimony as unprofessional conduct or the incompetent practice of medicine, they have the authority to discipline physicians who give improper testimony. The American Medical Association and other professional organizations and many physicians consider expert witness testimony to be the practice of medicine [25].

Because it is uncertain whether such disciplinary actions will be upheld in court, each state board should explicitly promulgate standards that define the standard of care for medical expert testimony or define the giving of improper testimony as unprofessional conduct. Moreover, it is not uncommon for plaintiffs in medical malpractice actions to hire out-of-state medical expert witnesses. Thus, many state medical boards are relatively powerless to discipline the conduct of out-of-state physicians or conduct that falls outside the practice of medicine. States should consider making provisions for granting temporary licenses for a specific purpose to regulate these out-of-state physicians.

Peer review by professional organizations

The leading court decision is *Austin v American Association of Neurological Surgeons* [22]. The following case summary demonstrates the feasibility and validity of an important means of professional self-regulation against unprofessional testimony.

The Professional Conduct Committee of the American Association of Neurological Surgeons (AANS) found that Dr. Donald Austin, a Detroit neurosurgeon, provided inappropriate and unprofessional testimony as a plaintiff's expert in a medical malpractice case and recommended suspension of his membership for 6 months. Dr. Austin testified in the underlying litigation that permanent damage to the recurrent laryngeal nerve of a patient during the course of an anterior cervical fusion procedure could only have occurred as a result of negligence on the part of the surgeon, and testified, "the majority of neurosurgeons" would concur with his opinion. The Professional Conduct Committee concluded that Dr. Austin was wrong in both respects. They held that the type of injury in the case was a known risk in such a procedure and something that all neurosurgeons know or should know. Whether Dr. Austin misrepresented the standard of care or misrepresented his expertise—either was grounds for disciplinary action. The AANS Board of Directors agreed and approved the suspension of Dr. Austin's membership. Dr. Austin attempted to resign during the pendency of his case before the Professional Conduct Committee, but the Board of Directors refused to accept his resignation until the case was completed, in accordance with the AANS bylaws. After Dr. Austin's suspension became final, his resignation was accepted [26].

Dr. Austin then filed a suit in US District Court alleging that (1) he was deprived of due process, a charge he later dropped; (2) the AANS program violated public policy by discouraging physicians from testifying for plaintiffs in medical malpractice cases; and (3) the actions of the AANS had sullied his reputation and resulted in a substantial drop in his expert witness income. The US District Court ruled in favor of the AANS. On appeal by Dr. Austin, the AANS was supported by an amicus brief filed on behalf of the American Medical Association, the American College of Surgeons, and the Illinois State Medical Society [26].

In writing the US Court of Appeals Seventh Circuit decision affirming the ruling of the lower court opinion, Chief Judge Posner praised the AANS Professional Conduct Program as a public service, writing that "this kind of professional self-regulation furthers, rather than impedes, the cause of justice" [26].

Chief Judge Posner went on to write [22],

> By becoming a member of the prestigious American Association of Neurological Surgeons, a fact he did not neglect to mention in his testimony in the malpractice suit against Ditmore, Austin boosted his credibility as an expert witness. The Association had an interest—the community at large had an interest—in Austin's not being able to use his membership to dazzle judges and juries and deflect the close and skeptical scrutiny that shoddy testimony deserves.

In January 2002, the US Supreme Court refused to hear a further appeal by Dr. Austin's counsel. The finality of the Austin decision stands today as the definitive court opinion supporting the right and, arguably, the duty of professional associations to discipline their members who engage in unprofessional conduct while testifying as expert witnesses.

Whether other associations will expend their financial resources to defend their "self-regulation" programs in court will be seen in years to come on a case-by-case basis.

Thoughts on expert witness reform

We deeply value expert information in most contexts except, ironically, in litigation when it is often regarded with a great deal of suspicion. Expert information is used by countless decision makers—from patients when they choose between medical doctors or between attorneys for legal representation, to Congress when it considers proposed weapons systems or monetary policy. In each case, the decision maker must come to terms with the need to act on the basis of information that he or she is not competent to fully understand.

Experts will always be needed for court procedures. Some critics maintain that expert witness testimony reform is needed. Is the source of evil the adversarial system (with free reign to promote partisan views)? Is the source of evil intrinsic to unprofessional partisan experts? Can the system, if unable to properly regulate physician testimony and attorney zealousness, be improved on to achieve its true purpose: pursuing justice for the litigants, regardless of their wealth and whether they are politically well connected?

Regarding new developments in expert testimony reform, there is an initiative sponsored by the "Common Good" called Specialized Health Courts [27]. Historically, this option of "expert jurors" (those who could best tell the facts), was developed by sixteenth-century English courts. Also, there is currently only infrequent use of an established practice of court-appointed experts, which has the potential to be expanded [28]. Such experts were nominated by the English courts dating back to 1299. In juryless courts, such as patent and admiralty courts, experts sat alongside judges, providing them with sought-after advice. With either option, if selected by the courts, experts could reasonably be seen as impartial.

The rise of the adversarial system created a third historical option of experts as witnesses [10]. The central feature of adversarial fact-finding is that the parties are entirely responsible for the factual investigation of a case. This third option encourages trial attorneys on both sides to tightly control the flow of evidence and thus maintain extensive power over the evidence, including the selection and preparation of expert witnesses. The multiple potential remedies for this ongoing mechanism are discussed in this article. A better future sees an alliance between medicine and law to provide needed expert witness reform, but this means that judges can no longer remain passive umpires.

Summary

Expert witness testimony is an important function of physicians. Without expert witnesses, a truly injured victim of medical malpractice cannot legally recover any monies owed to them. Expert testimony is used to define (opine) the standard of care, whether the standard was breached, and whether the breach caused the plaintiff's injury.

The nature of judicial decision making is to bring finality to litigation. The adversarial system is rife with factors that conspire against independent and objective expert witness testimony. These factors include selection and financial pressures, bias partisan preparation, and creating defensive postures to battle against vigorous "personal" attacks by the cross-examining attorney. Nonetheless, personal integrity and adherence to professional qualifications and ethical guidelines helps the expert maintain the "high ground."

Testimony that is unprofessional, faulty, and false is difficult if not impossible to regulate within the current adversarial legal system. Illegal

witness testimony, for practical purposes, is a nonevent; however, when unethical testimony is considered, more avenues for regulation are available.
One can potentially use or encourage state licensing boards and professional
organizations to discipline this type unprofessional conduct, ethics violation, and incompetent medical practice.

The medical profession has the right and duty to enforce standards to
protect the integrity of the profession. Most important, its procedure
must be laced with "due process" every step of the way to be beyond re-
proach. This practice is critical because lawsuits are likely to be initiated
against these organizations, and a defensible fact pattern makes for good
law and just outcomes.

Finally, although beyond the scope of the article, future policy-makers
need to reconsider the three options for experts in the court room (expert
medical courts, court-appointed experts, and experts as witnesses) and to
reconcile expert witness testimonial problems inherent in our adversarial
system with regulations/legislation to achieve independence and objectivity.

References

[1] Wecht CH, Koehler SA. Book review. J Leg Med 2005;26:529–34.
[2] Sanbar SS, editor. Legal medicine. 6th edition. Philadelphia: Mosby; 2004.
[3] AMA. Code of medical ethics. American Medical Association; 2002. 9.07 Medical
testimony.
[4] Amon E, Winn H. Review of the professional medical liability insurance crisis: lessons from
Missouri. Am J Obstet Gynecol 2004;190:1534–8 [discussion: 1538–40].
[5] Cruzan v Department of Health. Cruzan 497 US 261.
[6] Furrow BR, Greaney TL, Johnson SH, et al. Health law. St. Paul (MN): West Publishing Co;
1995.
[7] Revised Statutes of Missouri. 537.037. Emergency care, no civil liability, exceptions (Good
Samaritan law).
[8] Freckleton I, Mendelson D. Causation in law and medicine. Burlington (VT): Dartmouth
Publishing Company; 2002.
[9] Mueller CB, Kirkpatrick LC. Federal Rules of Evidence. Rule 401. Definition of "relevant
evidence". Boston: Little Brown and Company; 1993.
[10] Golan T. Laws of men and laws of nature: the history of scientific expert testimony in England and America. Cambridge (MA): Harvard Univ. Press; 2004.
[11] Gross SR. Expert evidence. Wis Law Rev 1991;1113–232.
[12] Kesselheim AS, Studdert DM. Characteristics of physicians who frequently act as expert witnesses in neurologic birth injury litigation. Obstet Gynecol 2006;108:273–9.
[13] Hand L. Historical and practical considerations regarding expert testimony. Harv Law Rev
1901;15:40–58.
[14] Ryan M. The adversarial court system and the expert medical witness: 'The truth the whole
truth and nothing but the truth?'. Emerg Med 2003;15:283–8.
[15] Executive Board of the American College of Obstetricians and Gynecologists. Qualifications
for the physician expert witness. Available at: http://www.acog.org/departments/download/
ExpertWitnessQualifications.pdf. Accessed May 2, 2007.
[16] ACOG Committee on Ethics. Expert testimony. Available at: http://www.acog.org/from_
home/publications/ethics/ethics116.pdf. Accessed May 2, 2007.
[17] Berlin L. Malpractice issues in radiology: bearing false witness. AJR 2003;180:1515–21.

[18] Sorrel AL. Doctor indicted over expert qualifications. AMA News 2007;19:11–2.
[19] Matson JV, Daou SF, Soper JG. Effective expert witnessing: practices for the 21st century. 4th edition. New York: Crc Press; 2004.
[20] *Daubert v Merrell Pharmaceuticals*, 509 US 579 (1993).
[21] *Giffin v Summerlin*, 78 F3rd 1227 (7th Dist US App 1996).
[22] *Austin v American Association of Neurological Surgeons*, 253 F3rd 967 (7th Cir 2001).
[23] Turner JA. Going after the 'hired guns': is improper expert witness testimony unprofessional conduct or the negligent practice of medicine? Pepperdine Law Rev 2006;33:275–309.
[24] Eitel DR, Hegeman RJ, Evans ER, et al. Medicine on trial: physicians' attitudes about expert medical witnesses. J Leg Med 1997;18:345–60.
[25] AMA Policy H-265.993. Available at: http://www.ama-assn.org. Accessed May 2, 2007.
[26] Pelton RM. Third annual health law colloquium: medical societies' self-policing of unprofessional expert testimony. Ann Health Law 2004;13:549–61.
[27] Rhoades D. Common good and Robert Wood Johnson Foundation to expand initiative to promote health courts. Available at: http://cgood.org/f-rwjf.html. Accessed May 2, 2007.
[28] Mueller CB, Kirkpatrick LC. Federal Rules of Evidence. Rule 706. Court appointed experts. Boston: Little Brown and Company; 1993.

CLINICS IN
PERINATOLOGY

Clin Perinatol 34 (2007) 489–502

Error Reduction and Quality Assurance in Obstetrics

Amos Grunebaum, MD

*New York Weill Cornell Medical College, 525 East 86th Street, Suite J-130,
New York, NY 10065, USA*

Malpractice premiums for obstetricians have increased significantly in the last decades, and this increase continues to be a major concern for most obstetricians.

Frivolous malpractice suits increase malpractice premiums, and many believe that tort reform is needed to eliminate these suits. In a review of 1452 malpractice claims, however, the vast majority of resources went toward resolving and paying claims that involved errors rather than toward defending and paying for frivolous suits. Most suits that involved injuries due to error resulted in compensation (653/889 [73%]), whereas most of the claims that were not associated with errors (370/515 [72%]) or injuries (31/37 [84%]) did not result in compensation [1].

If we are trying to decrease malpractice premiums, in addition to working toward tort reform and eliminating frivolous suits, it should be our goal to improve patient safety and outcome and reduce errors in obstetrics.

The Institute of Medicine report "To Err Is Human: Building a Safer Health System" [2] reported that errors in health care are a significant cause of death and injury; all health care professionals agree that patient safety is important and should be addressed by the overall health care system.

Efforts devoted to optimizing communication and collaboration among the various members of the health care team are equally important in promoting these principles of patient safety. This goal is supported by many professional organizations that have encouraged physicians to reduce errors and to incorporate elements of patient safety into their practices.

The American College of Obstetricians and Gynecologists (ACOG) Committee on Quality Improvement and Patient Safety [3] stated seven objectives to make obstetrics and gynecology safer:

1. Develop a commitment to encourage a culture of patient safety.
2. Implement recommended safe medication practices.

E-mail address: amos@grunebaum.net

0095-5108/07/$ - see front matter © 2007 Elsevier Inc. All rights reserved.
doi:10.1016/j.clp.2007.03.017   *perinatology.theclinics.com*

Improve legibility of handwriting.

Avoid use of nonstandard abbreviations.

Check for drug allergies and sensitivities.

Always use a leading zero for doses of less than 1 unit (eg, 0.1 mg, not .1 mg); never use a trailing zero after a decimal (eg, 1 mg, not 1.0 mg): "always lead, never follow."

Write down all verbal orders received and read back the order verbatim to the prescriber to ensure accuracy.

3. Reduce the likelihood of surgical errors.
4. Improve communication.
5. Identify and resolve system problems.
6. Establish a partnership with patients to improve safety.
7. Make safety a priority in every aspect of practice.

This article outlines an approach to improve patient safety in obstetrics and gynecology, with the goal to reduce errors in labor and delivery.

Collecting quality measures: identification and recognition of adverse outcomes, errors, and near misses

The first step in the delivery of safe health care should be to identify and study the patterns of adverse outcomes and causes of error occurrence. Identifying these patterns can help obstetrician-gynecologists adopt and develop safe practices to reduce the likelihood of system failures that can cause adverse outcomes [4,5]. Table 1 [6] lists patient safety indicators that were developed by the Agency for Healthcare Research and Quality. Organizations may modify this list to meet their individual needs. Collecting safety indicators from departments may be helpful to assess progress in error reduction and patient safety, although there is no uniform agreement on this benefit [7].

Joint Commission on Accreditation of Healthcare Organizations National Patient Safety Goals and Sentinel Event Policy

The Joint Commission on Accreditation of Healthcare Organizations (JCAHO) is an independent, not-for-profit organization that evaluates and accredits nearly 15,000 health care organizations and programs in the United States and maintains state-of-the-art standards that focus on improving the quality and safety of care provided by health care organizations.

National Patient Safety Goals

Departments should regularly review the National Patient Safety Goals, which are regularly established by the JCAHO (Table 2) [8]. Hospitals are regularly surveyed to verify their compliance with these goals.

Although many of these goals do not necessarily apply specifically to obstetrics and gynecology, it is important that each department knows the

Table 1
Obstetric patient safety indicators developed by the Agency for Healthcare Research and Quality

Indicators	Numerator
Complications of anesthesia	Discharges with *ICD-9-CM* diagnosis codes for anesthesia complications in any secondary diagnosis field per 1000 discharges
Death in low-mortality diagnosis–related groups	Discharges with disposition of "deceased" per 1000 population at risk
Foreign body left during procedure	Discharges with *ICD-9-CM* codes for foreign body left in during procedure in any secondary field per 1000 surgical discharges
Postoperative hemorrhage or hematoma	Discharge with *ICD-9-CM* codes for postoperative hemorrhage or postoperative hematoma in any secondary diagnosis field, and code for postoperative control of hemorrhage or drainage of hematoma, respectively, in any secondary procedure code per 1000 discharges. Procedure code for postoperative control of hemorrhage must occur on same day or after principal procedure.
Selected infections due to medical care	Discharges with *ICD-9-CM* code of 9993 or 99662 in any secondary diagnosis field per 1000 discharges
Transfusion reaction	Discharges with *ICD-9-CM* code for transfusion reaction in any secondary diagnosis field per 1000 discharges
Birth trauma—injury to neonate	Discharges with *ICD-9-CM* code for birth trauma in any diagnosis field per 1000 liveborn births
Obstetric trauma—cesarean delivery	Discharges with *ICD-9-CM* code for obstetric trauma in any diagnosis or procedure field per 1000 cesarean deliveries
Obstetric trauma—vaginal delivery with instrument	Discharges with *ICD-9-CM* code for obstetric trauma in any diagnosis or procedure field per 1000 instrument-assisted vaginal deliveries
Obstetric trauma—vaginal delivery without instrument	Discharges with *ICD-9-CM* code for obstetric trauma in any diagnosis or procedure field per 1000 vaginal deliveries without instrument assistance

Abbreviations: ICD-9-CM, International Classification of Diseases, Ninth Revision, Clinical Modification.

Data from Johnson CE, Handberg E, Dobalian, A, et al. Improving perinatal and neonatal patient safety: the AHRQ patient safety indicators. J Perinat Neonatal Nurs 2005;19(1):15–23.

most recent National Patient Safety Goals and, as part of the effort to improve patient safety, ensures that it adheres to these standards.

Communication and team training

The JCAHO requires that accredited organizations identify and respond appropriately to all sentinel events that are defined as an "unexpected occurrence involving death or serious physical or psychological injury, or the risk

Table 2
2007 Joint Commission on Accreditation of Healthcare Organizations National Patient Safety Goals

Goal	Description	Application area
Goal 1: Improve the accuracy of patient identification.	1A. Use at least two patient identifiers when providing care, treatment, or services.	1A. Ambulatory, assisted living, behavioral health care, critical-access hospital, disease-specific care, home care, hospital, laboratory, long-term care, office-based surgery
	1B. Before the start of any invasive procedure, conduct a final verification process (such as a "time out") to confirm the correct patient, procedure, and site using active—not passive—communication techniques.	1B. Assisted living, home care, laboratory, long-term care
Goal 2: Improve the effectiveness of communication among caregivers.	2A. For verbal or telephone orders or for telephonic reporting of critical test results, verify the complete order or test result by having the person receiving the information record and "read-back" the complete order or test result.	2A. Ambulatory, assisted living, behavioral health care, critical-access hospital, disease-specific care, home care, hospital, laboratory, long-term care, office-based surgery
	2B. Standardize a list of abbreviations, acronyms, symbols, and dose designations that are to be used throughout the organization	2B. Ambulatory, assisted living, behavioral health care, critical-access hospital, disease-specific care, home care, hospital, laboratory, long-term care, office-based surgery
	2C. Measure, assess, and if appropriate, take action to improve the timeliness of reporting and the receipt of critical test results and values by the responsible licensed caregiver.	2C. Ambulatory, behavioral health care, critical-access hospital, disease-specific care, home care, hospital, laboratory, office-based surgery
	2E. Implement a standardized approach to "hand-off" communications, including an opportunity to ask and respond to questions.	2E. Ambulatory, assisted living, behavioral health care, critical-access hospital, disease-specific care, home care, hospital, laboratory, long-term care, office-based surgery

Goal 3: Improve the safety of using medications.

3B. Standardize and limit the number of drug concentrations used by the organization.

3B. Ambulatory, behavioral health care, critical-access hospital, disease-specific care, home care, hospital, long-term care, office-based surgery

3C. Identify and, at a minimum, annually review a list of look-alike/sound-alike drugs used by the organization. Take action to prevent errors involving the interchange of these drugs.

3C. Ambulatory, behavioral health care, critical-access hospital, home care, hospital, long-term care office-based surgery

3D. Label all medications, medication containers (for example, syringes, medicine cups, basins), or other solutions on and off the sterile field.

3D. Ambulatory, critical-access hospital, hospital, office-based surgery

Goal 7: Reduce the risk of health care–associated infections.

7A. Comply with current Centers for Disease Control and Prevention hand hygiene guidelines.

7A. Ambulatory, assisted living, behavioral health care, critical-access hospital, disease-specific care, home care, hospital, laboratory, long-term care, office-based surgery

7B. Manage as sentinel events all identified cases of unanticipated death or major permanent loss of function associated with a health care–associated infection.

7B. Ambulatory, assisted living, behavioral health care, critical-access hospital, disease-specific care, home care, hospital, laboratory, long-term care, office-based surgery

Goal 8: Accurately and completely reconcile medications across the continuum of care.

8A. Implement a process for comparing the patient's current medications with those ordered for the patient while under the care of the organization.

8A. Ambulatory, assisted living, behavioral health care, critical-access hospital, disease-specific care, home care, hospital, long-term care, office-based surgery

(continued on next page)

Table 2 (*continued*)

Goal	Description	Application area
	8B. Communicate a complete list of the patient's medications to the next provider of service when a patient is referred or transferred to another setting, service, practitioner, or level of care within or outside the organization. Provide the complete list of medications to the patient on discharge from the facility.	8B. Ambulatory, assisted living, behavioral health care, critical-access hospital, disease-specific care, home care, hospital, long-term care, office-based surgery
Goal 9: Reduce the risk of patient harm resulting from falls.	9B. Implement a fall-reduction program including an evaluation of the effectiveness of the program.	9B. Assisted living, critical-access hospital, disease-specific care, home care, hospital, long-term care
Goal 10: Reduce the risk of influenza and pneumococcal disease in institutionalized older adults.	10A. Develop and implement a protocol for administration and documentation of the flu vaccine.	10A. Assisted living, disease-specific care, long-term care
	10B. Develop and implement a protocol for administration and documentation of the pneumococcus vaccine.	10B. Assisted living, disease-specific care, long-term care
	10C. Develop and implement a protocol to identify new cases of influenza and to manage an outbreak.	10C. Assisted living, disease-specific care, long-term care
Goal 11: Reduce the risk of surgical fires.	11A. Educate staff, including operating licensed independent practitioners and anesthesia providers, on how to control heat sources and manage fuels with enough time for patient preparation. Establish guidelines to minimize oxygen concentration under drapes.	11A. Ambulatory, office-based surgery

Goal 12: Implement applicable National Patient Safety Goals and associated requirements.	12A. Inform and encourage components and practitioner sites to implement the applicable National Patient Safety Goals and associated requirements.	12A. Networks
Goal 13: Encourage patients' active involvement in their own care as a patient safety strategy.	13A. Define and communicate the means for patients and their families to report concerns about safety and encourage them to do so.	13A. Ambulatory, assisted living, behavioral health care, critical-access hospital, disease-specific care, home care, hospital, laboratory, long-term care, office-based surgery
Goal 14: Prevent health care–associated pressure ulcers (decubitus ulcers).	14A. Assess and periodically reassess each resident's risk for developing a pressure ulcer (decubitus ulcer) and take action to address any identified risks.	14A. Long-term care
Goal 15: Identify the safety risks inherent in the organization's patient population.	15A. Identify patients at risk for suicide. 15B. Identify risks associated with long-term oxygen therapy such as home fires.	15A. Behavioral health care, hospital (applicable to psychiatric hospitals and patients being treated for emotional or behavioral disorders in general hospitals) 15B. Home care

Adapted from The Joint Commission. 2007 National Patient Safety Goals. Available at: http://www.jointcommission.org/PatientSafety/ NationalPatientSafetyGoals/07_npsgs.htm. Acessed July 19, 2007. © The Joint Commission, 2007. Used with permission.

thereof." According to the JCAHO, all organizations should be engaged in conducting "timely, thorough, and credible root cause analysis; developing an action plan designed to implement improvements to reduce risk; implementing the improvements; and monitoring the effectiveness of those improvements." A root cause analysis is a process for identifying the basic or causal factors that underlie variation in performance (including the occurrence or possible occurrence of a sentinel event) and focuses primarily on systems and processes, not on individual performance.

The JCAHO regularly publishes on their Web site a "Sentinel Event Alert" [9]. In the July 2004 alert "Preventing Infant Death and Injury During Delivery," the JCAHO reviewed, under the Sentinel Event Policy, 47 cases of perinatal death or cases of permanent disability that were reported to the JCAHO.

Forty of the cases resulted in infant death and 7 involved permanent disability. In reviewing the root causes of these sentinel events, communication issues topped the list of identified root causes (72%), with more than half of the organizations (55%) citing organization culture as a barrier to effective communication and teamwork (ie, hierarchy and intimidation, failure to function as a team, and failure to follow the chain of communication). Other identified root causes included staff competency (47%), the orientation and training process (40%), inadequate fetal monitoring (34%), unavailable monitoring equipment or drugs (30%), credentialing/privileging/supervision issues for physicians and nurse midwives (30%), staffing issues (25%), unavailable or delayed physician (19%), and unavailability of prenatal information (11%).

Because most perinatal death and injury cases reported root causes related to problems with organizational culture and with communication among caregivers, the JCAHO recommended that organizations do the following:

1. Conduct team training in perinatal areas to teach staff to work together and communicate more effectively.
2. For high-risk events such as shoulder dystocia, emergency cesarean delivery, maternal hemorrhage, and neonatal resuscitation, conduct clinical drills to help staff prepare for when such events occur and conduct debriefings to evaluate team performance and identify areas for improvement.
3. Review and apply the ACOG "Vaginal Birth after Cesarean Delivery Practice Bulletin"; the "Standards and Guidelines for Professional Nursing Practice in Care of Women and Newborns" from the Association of Women's Health, Obstetric, and Neonatal Nurses; and the American Academy of Pediatrics and ACOG guidelines for perinatal care.
4. Develop clear guidelines for fetal monitoring of potential high-risk patients, including nursing protocols for the interpretation of fetal heart rate tracings.

5. Educate nurses, residents, nurse midwives, and physicians to use standardized terminology to communicate abnormal fetal heart rate tracings.
6. Review organizational policies regarding the availability of key personnel for emergency interventions.
7. Ensure that designated neonatal resuscitation areas are fully equipped and functioning.
8. Develop guidelines for the transfer of patients to a higher level of care when indicated, if essential services cannot be readily provided per ACOG guidelines.
9. Use a standardized maternal fetal record form for each admission.

It has been suggested that team training improves communication and that the principles of "crew resource management" in medicine may affect the individual's attitude and therefore decrease adverse outcomes; however, there are different views of the impact that team training has in reducing errors in labor and delivery [10,11]. Even in aviation, the precise impact that crew resource management has on improvements in safety is uncertain [12].

Recently, a study reviewed the impact of team training on a list of certain adverse outcomes (the "Adverse Outcome Index"). The investigators concluded that the "training, as [it] was conducted and implemented, did not transfer to a detectable impact in this study. The Adverse Outcome Index could be an important tool for comparing obstetric outcomes within and between institutions to help guide quality improvement" [13].

Documenting events in labor and delivery

Good quality of care requires good documentation. In addition to improving communications among labor and delivery staff and to providing the right care, documentation of the right care is crucial. Thus, education about proper documentation is essential. Without adequate documentation, it is often difficult to show that medical care was appropriate.

Specific issues related to patient safety in labor and delivery

The following are common problems leading to malpractice suits. Every institution should create guidelines and provide education and training to address each of the following issues.

Fetal heart rate pattern interpretation

Failure to accurately assess and interpret a fetal heart tracing is among the top allegations in malpractice suits. Miscommunication among providers plays a major role in these allegations. Every institution should adopt a common language for fetal heart rate patterns, preferably the nomenclature developed by the panel of experts convened by the National Institute of Child Health and Human Development [14,15]. In addition, further training of all personnel in the interpretation of fetal heart rate tracings should be implemented. For example, the author's institution requires that all nurses and attendings get specific training and become certified in electronic fetal monitoring.

Induction and stimulation of labor

Oxytocin, dinoprostone, and misoprostol are drugs used use for induction and stimulation of labor and have been associated with diverse adverse outcomes such as uterine hyperstimulation and ruptured uteri. They are also disproportionally involved in adverse outcomes and malpractice suits. Institutions should develop protocols that guide clinicians in using these medications. These policies should address issues such as informed consent, uniform protocols, preparation of solutions and tablets, appropriate and safe dosing and titrations, and management when hyperstimulation occurs.

Vaginal birth after cesarean

Since the publication of the *New England Journal of Medicine* article on adverse outcomes with vaginal birth after cesarean section (VBAC) [16], there has been a significant decrease in VBACs in the United States. Patients contemplating VBAC should be informed of the potential complications and provide adequate written informed consent. Prostaglandins should not be used in women who have had a prior cesarean section and are undergoing induction of labor because of the significant risk of uterine rupture. Women who have had two prior cesarean sections without a prior vaginal birth should not have a trial of VBAC. The increased risk of uterine rupture in patients who received oxytocin with a prior cesarean section has led several institutions including Parkland Memorial to not allow the use of oxytocin in patients who have had a prior cesarean section [17].

Magnesium sulfate

Magnesium sulfate is among the most frequently used drugs used in labor and delivery, as a tocolysis and seizure prophylaxis in preeclamptic patients. There have been reports of magnesium sulfate–related deaths in labor and delivery due to medical errors [18]. Simpson [19] outlined suggestions to reduce maternal injury and death due to overdosage of magnesium sulfate:

- Use premixed solutions.
- Use separate solutions for bolus and maintenance.
- Use solutions with less magnesium.
- Use color-coded tags on lines.

- Have 1:1 nursing during first hour and 1:2 nursing during maintenance.
- Have a second nurse double check all doses and pump settings.
- During transfer, have both nurses together at bedside double check status, dosage, and so forth.
- Discontinue medication by removing line from intravenous port.
- Implement periodic magnesium overdose drills.
- Maintain calcium antidote in an easily accessible, locked medication kit.

Shoulder dystocia

Shoulder dystocia presents one of the true emergencies in labor and delivery. When there is injury to the mother or the baby, it often leads to malpractice allegations of failure to predict or perform the right maneuvers. All members of the labor and delivery staff should be versed in the recognition and management of shoulder dystocia, including McRoberts maneuvers, suprapubic pressure, episiotomy, Woods corkscrew maneuver, and delivery of the posterior arm. Fundal pressure should never be used with shoulder dystocia.

A shoulder dystocia drill is a practice run-through by a labor and delivery unit of a mock shoulder dystocia delivery. It is used as a teaching technique for all members of the obstetric team and should be considered by all labor and delivery units. The ACOG has produced a shoulder dystocia video (AVL 103) that describes and visually demonstrates a model shoulder dystocia drill. In addition, mannequins have been successfully used to train labor and delivery personnel in shoulder dystocia [20].

Maternal hemorrhage

Maternal hemorrhage is among the major causes of maternal morbidity and mortality in labor and delivery. Protocols to identify and treat maternal hemorrhage early on should be implemented by each labor and delivery unit. Attention to improving the hospital systems necessary for the care of women at risk for major obstetric hemorrhage is important in the effort to decrease maternal mortality from hemorrhage.

A good example of how to improve maternal morbidity and mortality was shown by one institution [21] that implemented process changes at the direction of a multidisciplinary patient safety team. These changes included a rapid response team and protocols for early diagnosis, assessment, and management of patients at high risk for major obstetric hemorrhage. With these changes, the institution showed a significant improvement in mortality due to hemorrhage, lowest pH, and lowest temperature. The investigators concluded that despite a significant increase in major obstetric hemorrhage cases, there were improved outcomes and fewer maternal deaths after implementing systemic approaches to improve patient safety.

Operative deliveries: forceps/vacuum

In deliveries involving a birth injury, doctors are more likely to be suspected as negligent when the baby is delivered vaginally compared with cesarean section [22], and operative vaginal deliveries such as forceps and vacuum are at the forefront of these malpractice suits. By Googling "forceps malpractice," over 50,000 citations are revealed, and 9 of the first 10 citations lead to malpractice lawyers' pages on which the dangers of forceps delivery are explained in full and in often graphic details. Thus, every operative forceps or vacuum delivery that is associated with any problem will likely lead to increased scrutiny and a potential malpractice suit. Patients should be informed during their prenatal visits about the potential risks of interventions during labor and delivery. Informed patient consent should be obtained before operative forceps and vacuum deliveries, with full disclosure of potential problems including maternal injuries after forceps such as vaginal and perineal tears, injury to the anal sphincters and subsequent anal incontinence, bladder and urethral trauma, and urinary incontinence. Newborn risks include injury to the head and face, including abrasions and skull trauma.

Thrombembolic diseases

Decreasing maternal mortality is a complex endeavor [23], and prevention of deep venous thrombosis (DVT) should be among the priority of all obstetric units because pulmonary embolism is among the top three postpartum causes of maternal death.

Patients at increased risk for DVT include women ages 35 years and older, black women, and women who have thrombophilia, prior DVT, lupus, heart disease, sickle cell disease, obesity, fluid and electrolyte imbalance, postpartum infection, cesarean section, and transfusion [24].

Recommendations for thromboprophylaxis during pregnancy and postpartum are usually stratified based on risks such as a history of thrombosis or the presence of thrombophilia. Others advocate prophylaxis for all postpartum patients.

Patient at risk for thrombembolism should be identified early on and prevention strategies implemented. Prevention strategies include early ambulation after a vaginal delivery and cesarean section, use of intermittent pneumatic compression for post–cesarean section patients, and heparin prophylaxis for those who have additional risk factors.

Summary

Young [25] emphasized the need to improve patient safety and listed the following seven points concerning patient safety:

1. Safety is not a disciplinary function.

2. Safety is a prospective and continuous function. It is a journey not a destination.
3. Discipline is secondary to safety, although it may be a byproduct of safety considerations.
4. Discipline is a retrospective, episodic function.
5. Safety thrives in an atmosphere of fellowship and good will.
6. Judgmental attitudes are to be avoided.
7. To err is human but, more important, inevitable.

These points underline that despite efforts over the last decade to improve quality and reduce errors in labor and delivery, we are still in the infancy of understanding the cause of these errors.

References

[1] Studdert DM, Mello MM, Gawande AA, et al. Claims, errors, and compensation payments in medical malpractice litigation. N Engl J Med 2006;354(19):2024–33.
[2] Institute of Medicine. To err is human: building a safer health system. Washington, DC: National Academy Press; 2000.
[3] American College of Obstetricians and Gynecologists. Committee on quality improvement and patient safety. Washington, D.C., Number 286, October 2003.
[4] Pearlman MD. Patient safety in obstetrics and gynecology: an agenda for the future. Obstet Gynecol 2006;108(5):1266–71.
[5] Grobman WA. Patient safety in obstetrics and gynecology: the call to arms [comment, editorial]. Obstet Gynecol 2006;108(5):1058–9.
[6] Johnson CE, Handberg E, Dobalian A, et al. Improving perinatal and neonatal patient safety: the AHRQ patient safety indicators. J Perinat Neonatal Nurs 2005;19 (1):15–23.
[7] Grobman WA, Feinglass J, Murthy S. Are the Agency for Healthcare Research and Quality obstetric trauma indicators valid measures of hospital safety? Am J Obstet Gynecol 2006; 195(3):868–74.
[8] The Joint Commission: National Patient Safety Goals. Available at: www.jointcommission. org/PatientSafety/NationalPatientSafetyGoals/. Accessed July 19, 2007.
[9] The Joint Commission: Sentinel Event Alert. Available at: http://www.jointcommission.org/ SentinelEvents/SentinelEventAlert/. Accessed July 19, 2007.
[10] Barrett J, Gifford C, Morey J, et al. Enhancing patient safety through teamwork training. J Healthc Risk Manag 2001;21:57–65.
[11] Grogan EL, Stiles RA, France DJ, et al. The impact of aviation-based teamwork training on the attitudes of health-care professionals. J Am Coll Surg 2004;199:843–8.
[12] Salas E, Burke CS, Bowers CA, et al. Team training in the skies: does crew resource management (CRM) training work? Hum Factors 2001;43:641–74.
[13] Nielsen P, Goldman MB, Mann S, et al. Effects of teamwork training on adverse outcomes and process of care in labor and delivery: a randomized controlled trial. Obstet Gynecol 2007;109(1):48–55.
[14] Electronic fetal heart rate monitoring: research guidelines for interpretation. National Institute of Child Health and Human Development Research Planning Workshop. Am J Obstet Gynecol 1997;177:1385–90.
[15] Intrapartum fetal heart rate monitoring. ACOG Practice Bulletin No. 70. American College of Obstetricians and Gynecologists. Obstet Gynecol 2005;106:1453–60.
[16] Landon MB, Hauth JC, Leveno KJ, et al. Maternal and perinatal outcomes associated with a trial of labor after prior cesarean delivery. N Engl J Med 2004;351(25):2581–9.

[17] Cunningham FG, Hauth JC, Leveno KL, et al. Williams obstetrics. 22nd edition. New York (NY): McGraw-Hill; 2005.

[18] Simpson KR, Knox GE. Obstetrical accidents involving intravenous magnesium sulfate: recommendations to promote patient safety. MCN Am J Matern Child Nurs 2004;29(3): 161–9.

[19] Simpson KR. Minimizing risk of magnesium sulfate overdose in obstetrics. MCN Am J Matern Child Nurs 2006;31(5):340.

[20] Crofts JF, Christine B, Denise E, et al. Training for shoulder dystocia: a trial of simulation using low-fidelity and high-fidelity mannequins. Obstet Gynecol 2006;108(6):1477–85.

[21] Skupski DW, Lowenwirt IP, Weinbaum FI, et al. Improving hospital systems for the care of women with major obstetric hemorrhage. Obstet Gynecol 2006;107(5):977–83.

[22] Sachs B. Is the rising rate of cesarean sections a result of more defensive medicine? Medical professional liability and the delivery of obstetrical care: volume II, an interdisciplinary review. Washington, D.C.: The National Academy of Sciences; 1989.

[23] Campbell OMR, Graham WG. Strategies for reducing maternal mortality: getting on with what works. Lancet 2006;368:1284–99.

[24] James AH, Jamison MG, Brancazio LR, et al. Venous thromboembolism during pregnancy and the postpartum period: incidence, risk factors, and mortality. Am J Obstet Gynecol 2006;194(5):1311–5 [Epub 2006 Apr 21].

[25] Young T. Presidential address: human error, patient safety and the tort liability crisis: the perfect storm. Am J Obstet Gynecol 2005;193:506–11.

ELSEVIER
SAUNDERS

CLINICS IN
PERINATOLOGY

Clin Perinatol 34 (2007) 503–508

Responding Professionally to the Liability Crisis in Obstetrics and Gynecology

Frank A. Chervenak, MD[a],*,
Laurence B. McCullough, PhD[b]

[a]Weill Medical College of Cornell University, The New York Presbyterian Hospital,
525 East 68th Street, J-130, New York, NY 10021, USA
[b]Center for Medical Ethics and Health Policy,
Baylor College of Medicine, Houston, TX, USA

The professional liability crisis affects virtually every obstetrician–gynecologist in the United States today. Attention therefore has been given appropriately to macro-level issues such as tort reform and insurance reform, to address this crisis at the system level. At the level of daily practice, constructive proposals have been made about improving communication, documentation, adherence to practice guidelines, consultation, and even weeding out bad doctors [1]. Not all system-level and practice-level proposals will be implemented, and those that are will take considerable time to have an effect. Meanwhile, as recent work stoppages in some states indicate, among obstetrician–gynecologists there is considerable frustration, anger, and sometimes even despair about the future of the specialty.

In such a time of crisis, it is not surprising that economic survival can become paramount for many obstetrician–gynecologists. Older physicians, for example, are considering whether early retirement is as financially attractive as or even more attractive than continuing to practice. Younger physicians worry that rising premiums for liability insurance may not permit a fiscally viable practice. Physician leaders wonder whether practitioners are entering a world in which there is no margin and therefore no mission.

* Corresponding author.
E-mail address: fac2001@med.cornell.edu (F.A. Chervenak).

0095-5108/07/$ - see front matter © 2007 Elsevier Inc. All rights reserved.
doi:10.1016/j.clp.2007.04.003
perinatology.theclinics.com

As a result of these responses to the professional liability crisis, economic and other forms of self-interest can become dominant and displace fiduciary professionalism from its central place in the moral lives of obstetrician–gynecologists. The purpose of this article is to provide readers with preventive ethics tools [2–4] to respond professionally in their own practices to neglected ethical dimensions of the professional liability crisis. The authors' analysis and proposals are based on previous work [5].

The physician as fiduciary of the patient

The authors base their ethical analysis on the medical ethics of Dr. John Gregory (1724–1773), a Scottish physician-ethicist who first developed the concept of fiduciary professionalism in the modern period [6,7]. Gregory did so to correct the dominance of self-interest in the highly competitive, market-driven world of 18th-century medical practice in Britain. Gregory's concept of fiduciary professionalism has three components. First, physicians should accept the intellectual discipline of science so that theories of health and disease, and clinical judgment and practice based on them, can be free of bias. Following Francis Bacon's (1556–1626) philosophy of medicine, Gregory called for what has become evidence-based medicine. Second, physicians should make the protection and promotion of the patient's health-related interests their primary consideration. Third, physicians should keep economic and other forms of self-interest in a systematically secondary position. The first component of fiduciary professionalism provides the basis of intellectual excellence in medicine, while the second and third are the basis of moral excellence in medicine.

Four professional virtues and their implications for responding to the liability crisis

Four virtues put the concept of fiduciary professionalism into medical practice and leadership [3,4,8]. Virtues are traits or habits of character that make judgments about moral obligations and fulfilling them routine, rather than a constant struggle.

The professional virtue of integrity

The first and most fundamental professional virtue is integrity. This means practicing medicine according to standards of intellectual and moral excellence. Gregory argued that integrity protects patients and rightly identifies the profound sense of professional wholeness and satisfaction that comes from a life of intellectual and moral excellence in medicine [6,7]. Integrity never should be compromised. Otherwise, physicians destroy the profession of medicine from within.

One of the best ways to ensure integrity is for physicians and physician leaders to create organizational cultures that support and reward adherence to high-quality, evidence based practice guidelines and other disease management strategies. Such an organizational culture discourages the arrogance of idiosyncratic clinical judgments and promotes humility in the form of being open to correction of long-standing or even cherished beliefs and practices on the basis of emerging scientific evidence and its careful application to improve clinical practice. It has been suggested that doing so might reduce the risk of malpractice litigation, an added bonus [9]. In other words, the pursuit of intellectual excellence both enhances patient care, by reducing unnecessary clinical variation and its risks, while at the same time promoting self-interest as a consequence of good patient care. There is a general ethical lesson here for physician leaders in response to the professional liability crisis: the best way to keep economic self-interest in its proper place and nurture fiduciary professionalism is to make self-interest a function of excellence in patient care, not an independent goal. Failure to do so will contribute to the destruction of fiduciary professionalism, which is not as robust as physicians sometimes like to think [10].

The professional virtue of integrity has important implications for physician expert testimony in malpractice actions (defense and plaintiff alike). Expert testimony always should be directed to the identification of the range of the standard of care, identified on the basis of the best available evidence at the time of the case in question. This approach will serve as an antidote to slanting testimony in favor of the party who has hired the expert. Failure to adhere to evidence-based standards in expert testimony egregiously violates professional integrity.

The professional virtue of compassion

The second professional virtue is compassion. According to Gregory, this virtue obligates the physician both to recognize when the patient is experiencing pain, distress, or suffering, and act promptly to relieve the patient [6,7]. Compassion prohibits physicians from burdening patients with complaints to them about the professional liability crisis, because doing so is not consistent with the obligation to relieve pain, distress, and suffering. Work stoppages that ensure that patients' urgent needs are met are less problematic, but only when they do not interfere with the individual doctor–patient relationship. In contrast, adding to the distress of elected officials who are unresponsive to serious social problems such as the professional liability crisis is a time-honored civic duty that can be fulfilled without violating responsibilities in patient care [11].

The professional virtue of self-effacement

The third professional virtue is self-effacement. Again appealing to Gregory, the authors point out that this virtue requires physicians to put aside and not be influenced by irrelevant differences with patients such as race, gender, sexual orientation, and socio–economic status [6,7]. Should a patient threaten to sue the obstetrician–gynecologist, he or she should not respond any differently in the subsequent management of the patient than as required by standards of clinical excellence. Similarly, the fact that the patient is a well-known plaintiffs' malpractice attorney should have no effect on the physician's management of the patient. Self-effacement is a major antidote to distorting bias in clinical judgment and practice.

The professional virtue of self-sacrifice

The fourth professional virtue is self-sacrifice, which requires the physician to take reasonable risks to self-interest in patient care [6,7]. The resurgence of life-threatening infectious diseases in the past two decades from such pathogens as HIV and hepatitis B virus (HBV) has resulted in physicians routinely taking risks to health and life in meeting patient care responsibilities. With the encouragement and role-modeling of physician leaders, physicians should remind themselves that while financial risks are real, they are not as important as risks to health and life and therefore should not be regarded as of paramount importance. Keeping economic self-interest in its proper, secondary place serves as a powerful antidote to economic conflicts of interest that can undermine fiduciary professionalism by introducing distorting, self-serving bias into clinical judgment and practice.

Unethical responses to the liability crisis

The professional virtues taken together expose as unethical strategies that physicians sometimes employ in the clinical setting to reduce the risk of litigation. Physicians should not engage in crepe-hanging, (ie, distorting the informed consent process by accenting potentially adverse outcomes of very low incidence to decrease expectations and the risk of litigation). This practice, which can occur in the surgical aspects of obstetrics and gynecology, violates the integrity of the informed consent process and self-sacrifice [12]. Similarly, if an uncertain obstetric ultrasound finding is found in the second trimester, a physician may explicitly or implicitly steer a patient toward abortion, to reduce the potential liability that occurs with the birth of a child with anomalies. This strategy violates the integrity of nondirective counseling and self-sacrifice. Lastly an obstetrician who performs an nonindicated cesarean delivery on a patient with the intent of reducing liability for birth injuries to the infant violates integrity, self-effacement, and self-sacrifice. It should be obvious that the professional virtue of compassion is violated in all three examples.

The need for supportive organizational culture

Expecting physicians to maintain fiduciary professionalism in response to the professional liability crisis on their own is unrealistic. A supportive organizational culture is crucial [8,13,14]. Physician leaders are responsible for shaping organizational cultures and therefore have a critical role to play in effectively addressing the ethical dimensions of the professional liability crisis. They should create organizational practices and policies designed to acknowledge and reward physician behavior based on the professional virtues [4]. Some behaviors, such as adherence to practice guidelines, can be measured reliably and assessed. For example, continuous quality improvement is a major preventive ethics tool for maintaining individual and organizational integrity. Physician leaders should be explicit about the preventive ethical significance of this and other management tools so they do not become subordinate to survival for its own sake.

Some behaviors, such as inappropriate counseling of patients, are not measured easily and assessed and present more formidable preventive ethics challenges to the physician leadership. There is no canary in the mine to warn a physician leader that the professional virtues and the organizational culture are in ethical peril from these hard-to-detect physician behaviors. The authors believe that strengthening the fiduciary professionalism of an organization's culture will strengthen individual fiduciary professionalism, especially in these hard-to-assess areas. Physician leaders should make it clear that maintenance of individual fiduciary professionalism is essential for maintaining organizational fiduciary professionalism.

Summary

An inadequate response to the ethical dimensions of the professional liability crisis is to focus only on system-level policy changes and therefore fail to acknowledge that the decisions of individual physicians and physician leaders are also essential for responsibly managing that crisis. The professional liability crisis needs not only a top-down but also a bottom-up response. The concept of fiduciary professionalism and the professional virtues that put it into practice should be used by physicians and physician leaders to create ethical best-practice models that can improve organizational cultures and therefore guide macro-level tort and insurance reform. This microlevel response, over which physicians and physician leaders do indeed have effective control, will serve as a powerful antidote to the increasing and ethically malignant dominance of survival and economic self-interest in individual, organizational, and public policy discourse and action.

A worse and ultimately ineffective response to the professional liability crisis is to give oneself over to anger and despair. This is a simple and seductive alternative. The reader, however, should remember the ancient wisdom, "Whom the gods would destroy, they first make angry."

References

[1] Queenan JT. Professional liability—some solutions. Obstetrics & Gynecology 2001;90(3): 365–8.
[2] Chervenak FA, McCullough LB. Clinical guides to preventing ethical conflicts between pregnant women and their physicians. Am J Obstet Gynecol 1990;162:303–7.
[3] McCullough LB, Chervenak FA. Ethics in obstetrics and gynecology. New York: Oxford University Press; 1994.
[4] Chervenak FA, McCullough LB. The moral foundation of leadership: the professional virtues of the physician as fiduciary of the patient. Am J Obstet Gynecol 2001;184:875–80.
[5] Chervenak FA, McCullough LB. Neglected ethical dimensions of the professional liability crisis. Am J Obstet Gynecol 2004;190:1190–200.
[6] McCullough LB. John Gregory's writings on medical ethics and philosophy of medicine. Dordrecht (The Netherlands): Kluwer Academic Publishers; 1998.
[7] McCullough LB. John Gregory and the invention of professional medical ethics and the profession of medicine. Dordrecht (The Netherlands): Kluwer Academic Publishers; 1998.
[8] Chervenak FA, McCullough LB. Physicians and hospital managers as cofiduciaries of patients: rhetoric or reality? Journal of Healthcare Management 2003;48:172–9.
[9] Ransom SB, Studdert DM, Dombrowski MP, et al. Reduced medicolegal risk by compliance with obstetric clinical pathways: a case–control study. Obstet Gynecol 2003;101:751–5.
[10] Rothman DJ. Medical professionalism—focusing on the real issues. N Engl J Med 2000;342: 1284–6.
[11] King ML Jr. Letter from Birmingham jail. In: King ML, editor. Why we can't wait. New York: New American Library; 1964. p. 76–95.
[12] McCullough LB, Jones JW, Brody BA. Informed consent: autonomous decision making of the surgical patient. In: McCullough LB, Jones JW, Brody BA, editors. Surgical ethics. New York: Oxford University Press; 1998. p. 15–37.
[13] Chervenak FA, McCullough LB. Professionalism and justice: ethical management guidelines for leaders of academic medical centers. Acad Med 2002;77:45–7.
[14] Chervenak FA, McCullough LB. The diagnosis and management of progressive dysfunction of health care organizations. Obstet Gynecol 2005;105:882–7.

ELSEVIER
SAUNDERS

CLINICS IN
PERINATOLOGY

Clin Perinatol 34 (2007) 509–513

Index

Note: Page numbers of article titles are in **boldface** type.

Moving?

Make sure your subscription moves with you!

To notify us of your new address, find your **Clinics Account Number** (located on your mailing label above your name), and contact customer service at:

E-mail: elspcs@elsevier.com

800-654-2452 (subscribers in the U.S. & Canada)
407-345-4000 (subscribers outside of the U.S. & Canada)

Fax number: 407-363-9661

Elsevier Periodicals Customer Service
6277 Sea Harbor Drive
Orlando, FL 32887-4800

*To ensure uninterrupted delivery of your subscription, please notify us at least 4 weeks in advance of move.